IF IT WERE JUST CANCER

A BATTLE FOR DIGNITY AND LIFE

Janette Byrne

VERITAS

First published 2006 by
Veritas Publications
7/8 Lower Abbey Street
Dublin 1
Ireland
Email publications@veritas.ie
Website www.veritas.ie

ISBN 1 85390 979 3
978 1 85390 979 5

10 9 8 7 6 5 4 3 2 1

Printed in the Republic of Ireland
by Betaprint Dublin

Veritas books are printed on paper made from the wood pulp of managed
forests. For every tree felled, at least one tree is planted, thereby renewing
natural resources.

Acknowledgements

I read the acknowledgements in books all the time but until I wrote *If It Were Just Cancer* I never realised the significance and necessity of this paragraph. For me there are a lot of people who were truly instrumental in getting my book to where it is now. My parents, who gave freely their love and support; my partner Declan, for his understanding and for his strong shoulder when the tears came; Graham, my son, for his humour and indifference to his mother's writing frenzies; my siblings, for their ongoing encouragement and pride; Ruth and colleagues at Veritas, for the chance to be heard; my friends in the little class of writers and a teacher without whose inspiration, assistance, kindness and patience *If It Were Just Cancer* would still be locked away in my mind and heart. Thank you Eithne for your friendship and unrelenting patience. The doctors and nurses who work every day in appalling conditions; I applaud you. And finally to those who are no longer with us in body but whom I felt were always with me in spirit on this journey of truth.

The new millennium has just arrived and is greeted by a world of expectations. I write from a place that feels so different from the one I knew. So much has changed around me, but, most of all, I have changed. I want to tell you everything and I don't know why. I feel compelled to do so in memory of the most wonderful women I have ever met — mothers, sisters, wives, daughters and friends. They were all something to someone and broken hearts move amongst us every day, struggling to move on and find some peace and normality. Children now deprived of the love of their mother; husbands and partners mourn the loss of a best friend and life companion. Daughters and sons missed by parents, who are left lost and racked with feelings of guilt as their lives continue and the young die. Friends worry if they had helped enough. Could their friendship have given more? Now it matters no longer. These wonderful people are gone from this life, but live on in the hearts and minds of those who loved them.

A world of memories floats around us, the only link when all else has gone.

Looking Back

February 2000

For over a year I had struggled with illness; visits to my doctor had become regular and embarrassing. When I was yet again feeling unwell I tried to ignore it, knowing the kind of comments that would greet my latest complaint: 'God you're always sick, you could do with a good tonic.' People were fed up with me – I don't blame them, I was fed up with me! Sometimes I became so frustrated I'd wonder why I bothered with doctors' fees when I was surrounded by people always ready to offer a diagnosis. And even when I did bother to visit the doctor it was always the same result: antibiotics. The magic drugs and our GP's answer, it seemed, to everything.

My doctor would listen but her distraction with the queue piled outside her door was painfully obvious. Like an unwanted guest, I rushed my visit, knowing that every word I uttered delayed her further. I felt that I was in some way responsible for everyone's impatience, as they coughed and spluttered, sitting trance-like or scanning the wall desperate to avoid each other's eyes. The usual Irish pleasantries were all but erased, replaced by zombies peeling through germ-riddled magazines that had been ripped apart by some child ignored by its mother, she too disheartened or ill to care.

I had had enough. I could take no more. The whole thing was bringing me down. I decided I would take control of my health: I would wash that old doctor superiority crap out of my mind and stop pussy-footing around, accepting the continuous 'get-lost' prescriptions – prescriptions for medication, it seemed, that was only useful at giving me thrush. I demanded, well, asked politely, for that coveted letter of referral to one of Ireland's esteemed specialists. I went with an optimistic mind: these were our experts, the peers of our medical world, nesting together in their distinguished Dublin clinics. These clinics would have been well out my pocket's reach for many years, but now the fee was not even a consideration: I would have sold my home if someone could clear my mind, dissolve the mistrust of myself forming like an unwanted tumour in my brain, always goading, whispering thoughts of worry through my whole being. The doctors say, 'You're not sick', and, of course, *they know*. Maybe people were right; maybe I just needed a good tonic or a good kick up the arse. I just wanted the draining, unrelenting worry to go away; I wanted to return to my normal health, something I had taken for granted too easily. I would do whatever it took to turn back the clock. I felt this was the last time I would have the strength to acknowledge the tiredness, neck swelling, breathlessness and the other niggling signs my body pushed forward for me to feel – for without a voice these signs were my body's only way to communicate, to say, 'Hello! I am sick! Is anyone listening? Please help!' But it is ultimately up to us to take time from our busy schedule and to listen to our bodies.

Through the coming weeks my health continued to deteriorate. In May I attended the doctor's surgery three times. The embarrassment of every visit outshone the last, as I tried to read the receptionist's face. Did she think I was a hypochondriac or maybe just a moan?

1 June 2000

It was June when I met the smoked glass clinic with its cunning attempt at feigning a cosy, homely atmosphere, disguised to lessen our dread, to make us feel safe and relaxed, all the while displaying respect for the esteemed consultants working behind each door. To me the clinic felt like a giant hive, its interior a mix of golden browns and honey, closed doors dotted along the circular corridors. But this was a hive where everyone seemed to work in secret and alone. I had an objective and here I sat, nervous and shaky, waiting to find some hope. Would I now get the magic tonic to restore my strength? Fear whispered thoughts of fleeing to my ears, but I sat firm. I had come this far; I would stay.

The professor 'oohed' and 'aahed' and looked down my throat and, after a short examination, I left with a possibility. I now had with me a referral for an ultrasound and a phone number for a speech therapist. The first was to check for thyroid problems. The second was … I don't really know! I was a bit confused on that one and, like most people, I left without clarity. However, I was calmed by the fact that he couldn't really see anything obvious wrong and at least I had the tests to focus on. I was in control now, no more messing around. Things were happening and soon I would know what was wrong with me. Maybe it was thyroid – I had lost a few pounds lately and it certainly wasn't from depriving my gob!

30 June 2000

Weeks passed and I attended another reputable clinic. My heart filled with gloom when I was informed that the ultrasound was clear. I decided against spending more money on a speech therapist. However, I did phone the esteemed clinic a few days later. An event of Murphy's Law invoked this act. You see, on the day of my visit my neck was not swollen but a few days later it was out in all its glory. I was angered by its timing and rang the clinic, asking the relevant secretary if I could call to see the professor for a minute, just to show him this unusual transformation. This was a bit naïve of me, I suppose, but then I ran a business and to me my customers were some of the most important people in my world. They put food on the table, fed my child and allowed me the funds to enjoy the pleasures of this life. But this was not the Ireland of old where a family doctor lived by his Hippocratic Oath. A time remembered so clear in my mind when many a doctor's fishing trip or golf outing was cancelled. Memories of nights when our GP arrived with bed head and pyjamas still warm under his suit stayed clear in my mind. Those were times when the whole road could be stricken by an outbreak of scarlet fever or measles, when money came second to health and well-being. But now it is the year 2000 when sometimes we can get so caught up in procedures and protocol with little regard for each other. I was, of course, politely informed I would just have to make another appointment. I was fuming. I wasn't asking for a free visit! I would have paid in full, over and over. How in God's name could I know when this body of mine would display its illness again? I decided once more to resign myself to the system and take the snail's pace journey, all the while trying to convince myself there was nothing wrong. I had a business to run, which kept me distracted by day. By night, however, when control slipped away, I found peace in prayer. It stopped my mind from wandering and I begged, 'Please God, let me be well. Please St Anthony, let them find out what is wrong.' Each morning I hoped I would wake to a new day, healthy and full of energy – and, you know, some days I did.

Finding Lumps

I carried on for another few months, visiting my doctor sporadically with sore throats and neck swelling. Most days I was still consumed with anxiety and worry. I struggled from bed each morning now with less energy than a ninety year old. I was weak from bone to brain and I had now discovered two lumps in my neck. After much persuasion I agreed with my partner, Declan, to attend the doctor yet again – but only if he came and explained he had forced me to go. At this stage the thought of even facing the receptionist again filled me with shame and embarrassment. But Declan lives with me; he loves me and was suffering too. He could see what was happening. He knew in his heart I was sick and his frustration was building as weeks and months went by and no answers were found. I knew I was so lucky to have him and I thanked God for his support.

I wrote those words 'discovered two lumps' in the previous paragraph so blasé but, as you might imagine, this was far from the truth of how I felt at the discovery. It is a lie with the weight of a mortal sin, for that moment, with one innocent touch to a place of discomfort, was to change my whole life forever. My heart pounded in my ears, the rise and fall of my breast increased like some unnatural trick, compensating for the panic pulsating through my body. Every breath was leading me further from control. Tears ran down my face as confusion muddled my thoughts, negativity bombarded my whole being and the pillar of reason in my mind crumbled apart.

September 2000

I arrived at the surgery to be told my doctor was going on leave and I would be seeing another doctor. Like a tape recording I repeated my symptoms, now with the added fear of these alien lumps in my neck. He explained that he wished to discuss my case with my present doctor before she went on leave and he would come back to me as soon as possible.

October 2000

Weeks passed and still no word from my doctor. During that time I did a good job convincing myself that if the doctor thought for one minute there was anything seriously wrong with me he would be on the phone straight away. Most days the pain at the base of my throat was unbearable and unrelenting and I felt really miserable. So, yet again, I attended the surgery. Another new face greeted me and, to my disgust and shock, I found the previous doctor had failed to even enter any notes of my recent visit in my chart. The new doctor seemed much more concerned and relaxed – obviously the stress of the crowded surgery had not got to her yet. And, thank God, she agreed with my request for a fourth referral.

November 2000

In the typical style of our chaotic hospital system nearly a month went by and I received no appointment. With desperation in my heart I faxed another letter of referral through to the hospital myself. The following week I received an appointment by return letter. At this stage, I felt such frustration, but mostly I was just very sad and worried.

December 2000

I went through Christmas and New Year in a haze, attending my doctor three days before Christmas day. On this occasion my wheeze had worsened. I remember sitting in my sister Pauline's house and someone saying, 'Shush, what's that noise?' Everyone went still. I listened also, ears attentive, but slowly as the room of eyes followed the sound they came to rest on me. I was embarrassed. My lungs were crying, but no cough or splutter would silence their voice. I spent Christmas at my parents' house and I recall catching their sneaking glances of concern. I remember feeling very emotional all the time – the slightest nettle and I would walk away, tears brimming. It was so weird – as if the worst thing in the world had happened and I felt it without even knowing its name.

January 2001

25 January 2001

The New Year brings with it my long-awaited appointment, this time to a Dublin public hospital. A very nice, gentle doctor carries out a needle biopsy. He also arranges for me to have some scans. When the biopsy is being done I am consumed with terror. I go into a trance-like state wondering have I always known this is where my path would eventually lead. Now will I be happy for results and answers? Things have shifted. I am eventually being taken seriously and with this my feelings are changing from frustration and anger in my struggle to be heard and believed, to fear and worry – they are now my new best friends and they will stay with me in my heart for what might lie ahead. With one tiny pinch of a needle there is no going back. My prayers are being answered. 'Please God, let them find out what is wrong.' Will I rue the day I uttered that plea?

As the days pass I pretend to cast the impending results to the furthest corners of the universe and get on with my life, but every day and night not one nanosecond goes by that I am worry free. I develop a rehearsed line for those around, an air of indifference entering my voice in response to their concern. What a charade I play and those close to me play it too. Plastic smiles stretch across our faces and all our true feelings are deep undercover, hidden in our hearts.

My results won't be available for two weeks. How will I survive this mental torture? How can they want me to wait? Haven't I already waited long enough? How can they do this to people? 'Okay dear, we're just going to check and see if there is anything sinister in these lumps, now bye bye, see you in two weeks or so and have a nice weekend.' 'Yeah sure, okay, I can do that. I'm a bloody robot!'

I am consumed with anger. My mind is a mess. My friend Instinct has brought me this far but now I no longer want to listen to her.

February 2001

The Nightmare Begins: 1 February 2001

I wake up and instantly I know there is something very serious happening to me. The swelling in my neck and face feels in full display. My body is screaming from the inside out. The bloating forces my eyes to close; my breathing rasps as my lungs struggle to operate. It's strange, I have become so used to the swelling, hoarseness and wheezing that even now I try at first to shrug them off. But not this morning; I am not being offered the choice; it feels as though my body is on a path of destruction. Declan and my son Graham have both gone to work. I could see Declan's concern as he left, making me promise that I would go to the doctor again and saying he would call me in a while. I knew there was no way I could sit in a surgery. Aside from the consuming weakness, I knew people would stare, unable to control their curiosity.

I struggle to the side of the bed and force myself to stand. At this stage I have no idea how I will look. I stagger to the bathroom, mapping my way through squinted, swollen eyes. I stand staring in the mirror, the reflection now a stranger's face, distorted, bloated and streaked with tears. The crying makes things worse as my lungs struggle to work. I remember as a child my father would dampen a cloth and put it to our eyes when we had cried. I sit now on the loo, damp cloth cooling my face, trying desperately to calm myself. I feel light-headed and start to worry. Will I make it back to my bedroom, to safety, to the phone? I need someone with me and it has to be soon. I am petrified.

I am very lucky that my parents live about ten minutes away and Declan works close to our home. I dial Declan's number and wheeze words of panic: 'Declan, I am really sick, I can't breathe!' Hanging up I dial my parents, repeating the same message. It seems like only seconds have passed when Declan comes through the door, galloping up the stairs four at a time with no idea what will greet him. He is shaking and I can read the fear in his eyes as he struggles to make sense of what is happening. He kneels before me searching my eyes for strength, willing me to tell him I will be okay. His voice shakes as he calls the ambulance.

Now that he is with me I feel much calmer and I begin to work at slowing my breathing. In the panic I somehow remember a yoga class I took and the instructions for times of stress. I have only ever truly practised these when late for an urgent appointment and stuck in a Dublin traffic jam. Now I am hoping their power will be enough for this time of great need. I take deep breaths, hold them, exhaling out, focusing on my breathing, repeating a mantra in my head, 'You will be okay. You will be okay. You will be okay'. Thankfully this is helping and my breathing is easing. I feel a gentle, soothing circle inside me. Things are calming slightly and with this come thoughts of madness. I want now in my crazy head to make light of this whole situation, to cancel the ambulance. I suppose part of me wants to ease the worry for Declan. I make my way to the bathroom for some space. I bend down ever so slightly and the room spins. My body continues to spin in dizziness. I call for Declan, terrified, as my sight fades in and out. I call to him in panic, over and over, 'I am going, I am going.' I don't know whether I mean dying or fainting, but one thing's for sure: all is not well.

My Mam arrives, consumed with worry for her child, as mothers will do no matter what age we are. And even in your thirties there is a wonderful safe feeling having your parents around when you are unwell. I suppose it's because all through my life they have made things okay and there is an inbuilt sense of security that comes over me.

The ambulance is taking forever and Declan is panicked as he stares at my face. I know now what stares back at him. It is as though I'm looking through a magnifying glass, eyes bulging, face distorted. Declan rings the ambulance again and chokes the words, 'Hurry, she can't breathe, please, hurry'.

Eventually they come charging up the stairs, apologising that they couldn't find the house. Well, in fairness, only in Ireland do the house numbers jump from 102 to 56. We live on a street where its residents could struggle to find their own home! My bedroom shrinks as three burly men gather inside, one peeping above the other's shoulder to take a look. My Mam and Declan back away, relieved, letting the experts through. 'Have you eaten nuts, seafood?' Someone was taking control. 'Yes to all of them, but for years.' I know where he's going – anaphylactic shock, an allergy that would show itself in this way. God, maybe, could this be it? I let my mind play with this notion and it seems like a wonderful solution to my year or so of illness. I try to remember had I eaten something different but, sadly, no and yet again I am robbed of an answer. Through all these questions my mind screams in fear, 'Just get me to the hospital!', a place I have only ever been to have my tonsils out at twelve and to give birth to my son twenty years ago. I just want to be surrounded by the experts and the tools of their trade, just in case. I feel at this moment that it is the only place I will feel safe. No one in this room can help me now.

The ambulance whizzes through the streets, siren blaring, stopping only for the idiot who won't move to let them through. Mam stares at me, her face a distortion of worry as I sit tossing from side to side. We eventually arrive at the hospital and I am despatched to the Accident and Emergency room. All prior sense of hope for a feeling of safety and security vanishes in an instant. The manic overcrowding makes me worry. Will I be lost among this lunacy, will I choke and die before I am even seen by a doctor? But then, let's face it, I have nowhere else to go.

My medical details to date are relayed to the attending nurse. I explain that scan results lie lingering in an unread file somewhere in the bowels of this chaotic hospital. As it happens the gods are smiling on me: the throat clinic which had arranged the scans and biopsy will be open at 2.30 p.m. today. I am sure it is with relief that the Accident and Emergency staff can wash their hands of me.

Again I play the waiting game. It is now 11.30 a.m. Time crawls when you can't breathe and fear is smothering you. Finally, the time comes and I am wheeled passed the waiting mass of queuing public. People's stares of curiosity follow me, I suppose calculating if I really deserve to skip the snaking queue. I am greeted by the clinic doctor's apologies. It seems I will be delayed again as they search for the scan results. They are having trouble locating them. (In a moment of madness I wonder if somehow those results are never seen and read will my life's path remain the same.) Eventually I get to see the boss and his team. The fact that I am seeing the main man makes me worry for my life. There are about four doctors surrounding me, asking numerous questions, and they are all ears and attentive in their listening. The scans, like large photo negatives, enter the room. I stare, my eyes never leaving them, knowing they hold the answer. My wait is nearly over.

The doctor is very kind. He includes us in their reading and for this I am glad – these are my insides, my vessels. He explains gently that there is cause for concern. The biopsy has shown negative cells and now the scans show a tumour staring back at us, all 11x8cm of it (about the size of a packet of cigarettes). It is still growing, crawling, choking, attaching itself to my windpipe. I ask for a glass of water as my lips seem to parch instantly. My body has a very unwanted guest. Now the job ahead is to see how it will damage me. Is it cancer free and friendly or is it a fiend of death here to take my life?

I sit in the wheelchair stunned; something is happening in my head: it is as if I go into emotional overload. Some sort of indifference takes over as shock consumes me and part of me shuts down. I go into a haze of drifting, being wheeled, led, injected, questioned, but all as if I have moved outside of myself and am looking in. I am informed that an urgent operation will be carried out – these visitors will be interrogated as to their intentions with my body – but it will have to wait until the next afternoon. Only then can they truly give an exact account of what is going on. I go back to Accident and Emergency feeling lonely and dishevelled, but very lucky when I see the same ashen faces, unmoved, their eyes glazed and dead. It is as though the chaos has got worse. I feel so grateful – at least I have seen someone and things are being done. That is, of course, if they can slot me in.

The speed at which everything is now happening adds to my fear; that and a visit from whom I suspect is a counsellor really has me confused. She speaks in soothing tones and I feel like screaming into her face, 'You have the wrong person, go away and check your files!' My head spins. Why is she here? Is she actually a counsellor? Has my fate already been decided? Have I missed something in the trance? Panic sees its chance and creeps in. I need to check with my Mam; she was there and she will remember what was said. But she has no hidden secret or clarity for me. My family huddle around me in a circle of fear; worry obvious in their eyes as they speak to this lady, their concerns eventually aired. We have lost so many close family members to cancer: three grandparents, two aunties and an uncle, the last two leaving behind young families. Life was robbed from them with so much left to do; young children were left without a mother or father. Will this be my fate? My son has never had a relationship with his father; will he now be denied his mother also? Thoughts present themselves in my head that I can't even contemplate. We will just have to wait and see what happens.

***

I watch as the staff rush about, weariness etched on their faces. Space, the enemy; patients, the catalyst to stress. The nurses are so busy they don't even have time to pop a head in to check for our toilet requirements, never mind to see if you have choked to death or been raped – a genuine worry for me as I lie hidden away in a tiny room with two strange men either side. I feel so weak and vulnerable, and in a situation I would never, ever put myself, even in full health. I try calling for attention but being away from the nurse's station makes it impossible to be seen or heard. I feel isolated and lonely. I feel terrified and sad.

Declan comes back to Accident and Emergency and stays the night on a plastic chair. He is unable to find any comfort, never mind sleep. He pleads with me to rest, to close my eyes and try to get some sleep, an act totally impossible lying on a trolley – a trolley only ever designed for human transportation, its gruelling lack of comfort a reminder that it was never meant as a bed for overnight occupancy. Even when I calm down and am just about to drift asleep someone calls out, slams a bin lid shut or cries out in anger or pain. The added torture of the treasured mobile phones shrills into the sickly night air. It is impossible. Sleep evades me as the chaos consumes me, drawing me into my new reality – a nightmare of indignity and discomfort.

I need to use the bathroom and I don't know if I am allowed up and about. Still in my flimsy nightdress and nightgown I pad to the toilet in my slippers. No one bats an eyelid. So I carry on my way to the nearest toilet. This is located outside at the casualty exit. I am surprised to see gangs of injured and ill, people staring vacantly, waiting for help. I know from the other side that there is already no room at the inn. My heart gives a pang of pity for the aged and innocent, fear etched on their faces. It reminds me of a scene from one of those old black and white war movies we watched as children. Blood splatters the floor as a bandaged head bleeds through; an old lady sits crying, with pain I suppose; and a girl vomits over and over in a bowl already too small to accommodate her lot.

The wind blows through the open doors, freezing me to the bone. My body shakes uncontrollably and my teeth chatter, I imagine, in a combination of cold and fear. I venture on to the toilet. It doesn't take long for me to realise the gender rule of ladies or gents is non-existent here, as the man waiting before me enters the ladies. I hug my panty pad to my body, trying to savour some dignity and privacy. A young lad lies on the floor, a needle ready to stick into his scrawny arm. Roars bellow from the other loo and the door opens with a belt. A burly, scruffy fella hollers out his complaints to the world. Through blurry eyes I watch him stagger away. I shake my head in disbelief at the bedlam everywhere.

Inside, the toilet stinks and I discover it is bare of any hygiene necessities. I thank God as a lady comes and offers me a tissue from her purse. The door has no lock and my stomach churns at the dirt of the place. I wish I could put a hand on either side of the wall so it could take my weight and I could hover above the loo, but I cannot bear to touch their filth. Instead I opt for perching half on, half off the toilet, my leg just barely making it as a doorstop. My heart thumps, expecting that some strange man will burst through and catch me, taking the last shred of dignity I possess. I leave flustered, disturbed but mainly disgusted that I am in a hospital and unable to do the basic action of washing my hands. I open the door, avoiding as best I can any real contact with the handle. As I pass the waiting mass I bow my head in guilt as envious eyes watch me pass through the coveted doors. I suppose they assume they will feel better once they pass to the other side. God! How disillusioned they will be. I feel pity for every single one of them.

Through the endless night I doze fitfully, every so often stirring in panic, checking my surroundings in a haze of confusion. Declan's eyes stare back weak, no longer able to pretend, his mask dropped, peeled away by weariness and worry. His face shows his fear and sadness for the day to come, but both of us also long for its arrival, knowing that at least it will take us from the nightmare of Accident and Emergency, making space, we know in sadness, for the next poor unfortunate who will fill my trolley.

**

I don't remember the dawning of this day. Determining day or night is impossible in Accident and Emergency. Fluorescent lights pierce my eyes for endless hours; no windows to view the outside world and the unrelenting chaos that is Accident and Emergency confuses me. I am in a nightmare and there is, it seems, no waking. In the afternoon I am eventually moved from Accident and Emergency to a ward. The comfort of a bed is unbelievably welcome. If you have been there you will know what I mean. It is as though the mattress is three-foot thick and the peace of a ward is like switching from the Naas Road Dublin to Main Street Dingle in winter.

It seems I have only stretched on the bed when a young, friendly male nurse comes for me with a trolley. He is, I find out later, Filipino. Unfortunately his English is not great and communication is difficult. Normally I would relish the chance to learn about a different culture but today I am in no mood for this effort. Nurse produces a green gown for me to wear, leaving me concerned for my modesty and unsure as to whether knickers and bra should stay or go – a minor detail, but one that is unknown until you have experienced an operation. I'm sure that to the medical staff we must seem like idiots, but in my mind they will not be operating lower than my chest so maybe I can leave on the underwear. It took me time to clarify, but it is made clear to me that I should be naked but for the gaping gown. One hurdle jumped but now the wall: how can I explain to a male nurse who struggles with English that I have my period so I need my knickers and there is no chance he is getting them.

You might think that at this stage I shouldn't care, but I have three sisters and for years as children we managed to dress and undress without ever displaying breasts or other private parts. The cold of winter would bring a great excuse as we hid under our blankets – Houdini would have been proud to call us his own! I don't even think I really saw my own bits until I had my first holiday and had space and privacy to have a good gawk! But today I clamber onto the trolley – set, it seems, for a giant – feeling like a clown entertaining the bored patients with my antics, as I display for all knickers and bare back. The hospital routine is alien to me and I silently pray it will stay that way.

∗∗∗

Theatre, a place I do not know, new ground, and I observe it now on the flat of my back. I try to control my eyes, curtailing their curiosity. What will I see? Some alien cold steel tools used for God knows what, their image enough to send me into a panic. I am brought first to a prep room. Porters waltz in and out, slagging each other, laughing loudly, a welcome distraction for me. I wish I could be them, working away, their time here controlled by a clock; mine now controlled by destiny.

A nurse arrives. I am told I am in a queue and my time slot is not yet free. She leans close whispering calmingly to me. 'Let's do some breathing exercises pet, in through your nose, out through your mouth. In, out, good girl.' She is brilliant. If nothing else it helps pass the time. Her own breathing sounds fierce and I suspect asthma. I can't help wondering if this is a ritual she carries out for every poor unfortunate or if my eyes are betraying my fear. Or maybe I have just found a kind, caring nurse who has been here herself and knows from experience the horror I feel. For whatever it is that inspires her, I am grateful and it eases my mood. I get the sense the other nurses think she is mad, as they stand by their patients also waiting, making stilted, mundane conversation. But I am glad she is mine. An angel sent to ease my fear. Eventually another nurse joins us and more serious things are discussed. Kind Nurse wishes me luck and off I go. My trolley is pushed through the theatre doors and my past is left behind, swinging in their breeze. I am wheeled on, moving towards a future never logged in my dreams and aspirations and I know one thing is for sure: there is no going back.

'Hi Janet. How are you today? We are just going to pop a mask on your face and we will need you to take deep breaths … good girl.'

I hear faint and confusing words:

'No Janet, now stop! We have to do it, stop. Stop! Someone hold her hands!'

I thrash and pull. I have woken up during the operation. Is this meant to happen? What is going on?

My next memory is being back on a corridor. It is a dark, old building. I can see my family: Mam, Dad, everyone. They are a distorted image. I struggle to focus on their faces. There's

Graham, my son, and Declan – they seem so far away. In my mind I speak, 'Come nearer, please, nearer.' My brother is saying something. What is it? I wave to everyone, channelling all my energy to my hand but all that moves is my finger. I look at it. Something is attached. It is so heavy. I am smiling. I am happy they are all here.

***

Intensive care

I wake frightened. Where am I now? I can see a man. He has a huge steel contraption around his head. God, he looks like death. I smile and wave. No response. Where is this place? A nurse appears. She smiles and talks. She is young and pretty. I respond. A gurgle comes from somewhere. Is it me? What is going on? There is something down my throat. I cannot speak. I want to scream. My eyes fill. What has happened to me? She soothes me with her voice. I am tired and I doze. I wake. Two nurses are washing me, I am embarrassed – I still have my period but I haven't the energy to care. I doze. I wake sporadically. My whole body burns, I need to cool down. I try to get attention with my eyes – every other muscle in my body seems to have frozen. I hand-signal a pen and paper. I write words: 'shock', 'afraid', 'water'. The nurse returns. I realise she is always just a blink away and that comforts me. The water warms so quickly, but she returns over and over, ice and water cooling me. I drape a cloth across my head; the icy water runs down my face and neck soaking me. I love it. It is my only sense of being.

The nurse speaks to me: 'You are in intensive care. You have a tube down your throat.' Terror rises within me but I never look, I do not turn in observation, fear keeps me fixed staring straight ahead. I sense that people are on either side of me. I never hear them speak though. It is a ward of silence broken only by the workings of the monitors. The human presence is always felt but never seen. I signal to the nurse that I need the pen again. I need interaction. I remember with immense clarity the instrument that wrote my words, my instrument of communication, my channel of fear and hope. I remember when I was a child seeing a teacher with one of these pens and wanting one so bad. Its different options of blue, black, green and red seemed so interesting to my child's mind and here I have one, its coloured fluid flowing as my lifeline. I look now at my notes and, like the child, curious and adventurous, I have tried all the options. My notes, a mess of shaky writing but a glimmer of hope shadowed in the collection of gaudy colours.

Days and nights drift, I have no awareness. I just assume nothing changes, time no longer exists. But today there is something different. People are coming from my left. I wait. I hear their steps and confused mumbles. They are crying, considerate muffles of pain, and my mind makes sense of it: someone has died.

Nurse tells me my family are outside and have been there all along. My mind struggles to comprehend, confusion clears, I write again, 'Big family, just my Mam for a min.' I don't remember if we spoke and but for this note I would not know she had been. Graham, my son, is my first visitor. He kisses me and his whole being shakes. I feel so sorry for him, a man now, unable to shed his tears. I know he has my family, Declan and his own girlfriend, Alison, for support and I hope he can find with them the space and ease to cry. I cannot imagine what it is like trying to make conversation with me. I nod occasionally and stare into his face, trying to answer with my eyes questions that need more than a nod of acknowledgement. I write with the little energy I have: 'I got my throat blessed today.' A nun had come. At least this is something positive and a topic for conversation.

***

I know now it must have been so hard for everyone to see me: drips, machines, tubes, stitches and the long wait. Three days to seal my fate. Hours that fly by unnoticed in their normal busy lives now tick, ticking away in slow motion, watched constantly by all in aggravation and despair, while I lay unaware of their nightmare. Every minute, every second brought hope to my family as they waited outside, longing for any snippet of news, any change in my well-being, good or bad. They watched the door every time it moved. Sometimes I caught a glimpse of their smiling faces as they peeped in, trying to catch sight of me – and what a sight! I lay there unmoving, a mess of wires and tubes tangled like ivy coiled round my head. This was the touch-and-go stage where every second tallies your fate. It seemed there is no reasoning possible in the human brain, no emotion to help understand or rationalise what was happening as a barrage of confusion attacks your mind and minute by minute I struggled to make sense of everything, but I doubted I ever truly would. So far we were still blessed, I still survived, lingering in that hidden, silent world while the hospital chaos carried on around us. Close by, other families who were not so fortunate left. Their lives were now shattered. Their days ahead filled with the despair of funeral arrangements, leaving those behind in the hospital embarrassed but grateful for every moment they remain, always hoping their nightmare will end with a happy resolve.

***

Diagnosis

Today they come together, strong and precise, a gathering of the clan. They assault my ears with words I cannot bear to hear, leaving me wondering if some drug has made me go crazy – like the time I tried some marijuana so strong that it messed my mind enough to scare me off it forever! Direct words spoken in serious tones:

'You have cancer.'

I am unable to utter the words that are screaming in my brain. 'What? Stop! Stop. No! No! I can't cry. I will choke. Don't make me cry. Stop! Stop!'

'We will have to start chemotherapy straight away. Your tumour ...'

Fading words now, making no sense, 'Blah, blah, blah ...' I shake my head ... 'No! No! No!' Tears are flowing.

New day. New night. I don't know. I no longer care. Someone comes and inserts a needle. My chemotherapy has started. He is friendly and a little sad for me, I feel. I write: 'How long are the treatment sessions and will I be sick with the tube in?' I know in my heart and lungs that I will breathe alone, if only they would take this tube out. Again I write, 'When will the tube be removed?' They talk above my bed. A muddle of words, explaining that they are unsure how it will be if they remove the tube, they may have complications. I want to scream, 'I will be fine!', but instead I just stare ahead and wait. Hours pass, doctors come and go and each day I bore them with my repetitive written requests: 'Please can you remove the tube?' and, amusingly, 'When can I eat or drink?' Well, I always loved my food!

My Intensive Care scribbles

First Day I WAS AMITTED
Swollen face ALLERGIC Reaction
Lost Breathe LAST THURS
By Ambulance

Thank you

WATER TO WARM
please   Soarry
I'm very shaky Today

when can I Have a drink
OF WATER

Only family & Declan my boyfriend

can I get ligt

Am I ~~Having~~ Having a Relaxant

PLease

Good Night

yes - 1 min very Tierd

HEAVY   THROAT SORE
         very Tierd

Cold WATER please
1 might be a
          sleep.
SAY good night

Thank You

MAM - FOR a MIN - CANT get lipso

High Dependency

I am moved now to High Dependency. I am so tired. I have no memory of the tube being removed. I am okay, just so weak. This ward is brighter but still so silent and peaceful. People stare, eyes glazed, too ill to move a muscle, too frightened to test their capability. There is a nurse's station with three nurses. I ask for a magazine, I am restless. It is the habit of reading every night that makes me ask. The magazine weighs of lead and my eyes have no will. I give up, but the comfort of this paper and its stories brings a sense of normality. I feel part of the outside world just for one moment. I doze fitfully. I have no comprehension of the reality for my family, outside, day after day. They are exhausted with worry and lack of sleep. Patience stretched to the limit in a muddle of emotions. I am not capable at this moment of any concern for them. I am incapable of any emotion.

My next memories are of being shifted to a single room. I am in a wheelchair, my whole being has seized up. My motor and batteries have died. All energy has drained from my body. I know now they want to leave me alone but I'm having none of it and cry, begging them to let Declan sleep near me – wherever, I don't care. I have no real thoughts about the logistics of this and the fact that this is a public hospital or, if I do, I don't give a damn! I am so upset and afraid, weak and distressed. It is eventually permitted and Declan sleeps the night on the floor. A sense of comfort comes over me and I relax and sleep. I have only sporadic senses of being and awareness. I assume some little potion is concocted to protect me from the pain and fear.

The next day I am moved to a public ward. I lie flat, restricted by tiredness and lack of will. I see little but for a lady with a bandanna and a young girl with patchy hair. Her eyes seem to portray contempt and I feel they must mirror my own. I hear roars over and over, screeches like a wild animal in pain.

I look around, fearful of what I might see, but needing to know. It is another young girl, unwell since her birth, her only form of communication alien and frightening to us. Her screams unnerve me. I feel so terrified and vulnerable.

My family come and go in turns as I lie wasted in my bed. As the days pass the drugs clear from my brain and awareness filters slowly in, releasing snippets of information for me to take on board and deal with as best I can. I have not spoken to my family about my cancer yet and denial sets in. I don't want to be on this ward with these sick people. 'Why am I here? Someone please take me home.' I am so weak, yet I must make the effort. I struggle slowly, aided, to the toilet, a snail's pace journey of fear. My head spins. I dare to look in the mirror. My face is a grim distortion. I turn away indifferent to its form; I don't give a damn.

Doctors arrive, white coats flapping. Professors followed by their team who hang on their every word, hoping someday they will command the respect with which their superiors are greeted. Beds are made, patients propped and cleaned, fresh air blowing through the ward with no regard for its occupants. And we return to our duty as sick people with a possible death sentence hanging over our heads, waiting for it to tip one of us ever so lightly, letting us know we are the chosen one. 'No, not me,' I want to scream. 'Get lost! Leave me alone! What did I do wrong? I've been a good person! I don't deserve this – it's not fair!' But instead I remain silent. I want so much to live. I have a wonderful life, a child I adore, a kind, caring partner and a family who love me to bits.

But I refuse to say, 'Why me?' Why anyone? What is the answer? No one seems to know. Well, who would? All the patients around me are looking for the same answers. Who else might have some insight? Maybe a counsellor, if there was one available. But what would they do but repeat soothing words they have learned on a course somewhere far removed from a cancer ward and its patients? No one has the answers I need. Why this horrible disease? Why now? Why?

***

Today I am taken for a walk along the corridor by the physiotherapist. She instructs me how to move again. I assume the operations, the shock, along with chemo and the stitches in my neck have all drained my legs of any strength. In my wildest dreams I could never, ever, have envisaged this happening to me. Apparently I need to straighten up, but mostly I need to walk alone. But I am afraid, afraid of everything. What if I fall and trip, burst my stitches or break a bone? Only last week I was a tall, strong woman whose work was very physical and here today a baby, dependent, unable to even stand alone. I fear that I know now what lies ahead when I am old and fragile – all life's energy will be sapped from my bones – and it frightens me. Maybe it would be best if I didn't make it after all.

I lie awake listening to the laboured breathing of the elderly lady sleeping three feet away and I feel like a child scared in the gloom of night, wanting her mammy for comfort. The ward is in darkness but for a distant glimmer of light and its glow eases my mind. I am restless. I toss and turn wondering if everyone else sleeps or if we all lie lonely, staring silently into a void of darkness, longing for health and normality. I have always said my nightly prayers since childhood, more out of habit than devotion. But I pray now into the lonely night. I beg St Anthony to help me, to guide the doctors and help them find the right cure. I implore Our Lady as a mother to protect my son and let me live. 'God, I know you are busy and people beg of you every minute of every day but please help me. I am too young to die. Give me a chance.' The tears flow and I feel human again and with any remaining will I plead and plead. I sense the presence of someone. I close my eyes and an old friend long gone from this world is there. He holds my hand and hushes my cries. He tells me I will be well and to believe this with all my being. I grasp his hand, warm and strong. I look to my right. A woman I loved as a child, a kindly neighbour, who was always full of mystery and stories, with the heart of an angel, sits now, silent, and through them both I know now: I will be okay.

***

9 February 2001

I am allowed home for a few days – it seems like a year has passed – but I must soon return for my second session of chemotherapy. I try to find some level of calm in the disorder of my feelings. I brace myself for my journey ahead. I am wheeled to the exit. Declan helps me to the car. I feel I have already completed the marathon and the race has not yet begun. I stare at everything anew. My life has changed and I view this world with eyes of wonderment. I want to shout to the streets, 'Watch your back, be careful, enjoy yourself, love life and each other. Don't worry, and don't work so hard.' I want to pass on this vital information to warn everyone. 'What's important is under your nose. Please open your eyes!' People continue about their day, oblivious to my jealous eyes gawking at them as they go about just being, living, breathing – doing normal things like running, laughing, taking a bus, eating lunch, walking close and happy together. All the things I took for granted ten days ago have now slipped through my feeble fingers.

It has been decided I should stay with my parents, that I should not be alone. I am content with this decision. Reason tells me I could not manage on my own – even if I had the will, my body does not have the strength. My parents are happy to have me and I am welcomed with the embrace of love.

I wake early in the morning. I am confused by my surroundings, a regular feeling when I wake now. It's as though my life has been kicked off kilter. Everything confuses me. There is silence in the house. I assume my father has taken the phone of the hook. It would normally be ringing from early morning with his business demands. I feel guilty for the nuisance I am in his life: pregnant at nineteen and now this. I shake the misery from my heart and struggle to the day ahead.

I want so much to wake again and find this was a nightmare. I would sigh with relief and spring from my own bed with delight for my day ahead. But instead I accept my lot and steady myself for the world. I find my brother-in-law, Pat, sitting alone at the kitchen table. A man of many words and a joker, but today he is lost for words. I read the sympathy and sadness in his eyes and I see the softy who is usually hidden behind a roguish exterior. We do the usual pleasantries and I feel for him, uncomfortable with me, and again I hate this world that has changed everyone. Why can't things be as they were before? I cannot bear this. It hurts too much.

Pat asks how I feel and I suppose trying to make things normal in some way, I joke, 'I am grand Pat, but Jesus I had a terrible nightmare.'

And he replies, his voice loaded with concern, 'That's awful, what was it?'

'Yeah! It was awful. I dreamt I had cancer!'

I feel worse – the joke didn't work. The air is dense with awkwardness. I see Pat stuck for words, both of us out of our depth, and I want to run and run and never stop.

***

I do little but lie about, useless to anyone. I want to laugh, to smile, but with reason. I want the people around me to be content and happy, no pretences just to make me feel better. I want it for real, the way it was before. I wake early and have slept restlessly. I look in the mirror and what reflects is the face of a stranger. Janette has truly left the building! I see dead, vacant eyes, sparkle extinguished by fear or medication. I see skin no longer rosy and fresh, but pale and drawn. Half moons of grey now lie beneath my eyes. My hair once glossy – and a crown of pride – is now dull, limp and dry. 'Oh my God, what is to come?' I don't think I can bear to know.

Today I have a rash. I am informed by phone to come in to the hospital and not to worry. They tell me it is probably from the medication. I attend the day ward.

Over the coming days I go through lots of different phases. First, I don't want to know anything. Ignorance is bliss. I don't want the C words used around me. I don't want anyone to say cancer or chemotherapy. I make up silly names for my chemotherapy, calling it my 'jungle juice'. I suppose I think if the words are not said it won't be real and somehow I will make it through this whole ordeal in fantasy land.

I have always hated taking tablets. The most I have ever taken was a painkiller for a headache or an antibiotic. Now here I am being pumped with God knows what and praying every day that they have selected the right cure for me, begging for my life and that these strangers will make me well again. My life is consumed now by a void and to fill it I need reassurance and the words, 'You will not die'. I long to hear those words and I am sure my doctor longs to say them. But I have to wait until my chemotherapy is finished to find out my fate. I am so terrified, I feel close to insanity. It is unbearable.

Losing more than just hair

I feel so ugly, my hair going in places, found now in the light of day like a strange pattern spread on my pillowcase or clumped in a mass blocking the plug hole in the shower. All sense of confidence slowly slips away, day by day. It has become unbearable. Bald patches like crop field markings spread around my head. Every natural touch, flick or scratch thins it some more and gradually, as the hours tick by and the chemo seeps further in, diluting my blood, the change can no longer be hidden and so begins the drug-induced transformation of my being.

I sit with my son Graham and a coffee. As we chat I run my fingers through my hair without a thought, only to retrieve a clump of waste. I hold it in a fist, hidden. It is a natural motherly reaction to protect my son from this sight, protecting him from my pain, my sadness. I continue chatting, never once missing a beat in our conversation. And then a realisation sets in: this is stupid; I cannot continue like this. So I make a painful decision. My hair must be shortened. I am disappointed, as I have spent months letting it grow, going through that horrible long/short stage. My hair is the longest it has been in years and I am finally getting to the stage when I can tie it up. But now it doesn't matter. Vanity no longer has a place in my world. I cannot bear the irritation and mess, so it must be cut. But who can I ask?

I couldn't bear a visit to the hairdressers. All the eyes focused on me. Having to play let's pretend. Neighbours' words of encouragement and sympathy rained on me in public. Even the thought is too much. I think of Anita, not just a hairdresser but a family friend. I know her father also has cancer. She will understand and I will feel comfortable with her. Will she mind? That is the question. Of course Anita says 'Yes'.

I sit in Declan's Mam's kitchen. Anita tries to make some shape or style from a scatter of hair. It is futile, a hairdresser's nightmare. She does the best she can but no hairdresser could make any style from a balding, patchy head, where every draw of the comb adds to the growing pile of hair on the floor. I look in the mirror. My head is a mess of dry, patchy clumps. It was unfair to have asked and I see now it could have been harder for Anita than anyone else; I know it was an impossible task. I am just prolonging the torture. Two hours later I face the truth: I must shave it all off. I know in my heart it will relieve the ongoing mess and stress that this slow loss is bringing. I have crossed another bridge.

I ring my friend Ann Moloney. She arrives with a head razor. She has only ever used it on her son and she is very nervous. I pretend it's fine, no problem – it's just hair after all. I try to convince even myself that, in the bigger scale of events, this is nothing – hair grows back, so move on, just take it in your stride – and I smile and joke as if nothing is wrong. My hair clumps to the floor and my stomach churns at a loss so painful and so sad I would never have imagined. I find that as I sit there surrounded by my sisters, friends and mother I feel detached, out of body and in this surreal time I face a new decision and my mind struggles with disbelieve. This can't really be true. But my mouth speaks to the room words, automatic, robotic, shocked words. Yet the obvious next step: 'Should I get a wig?'

This prompt is taken and discussion begins in earnest as to what might be the best option for me. I am reminded, for whatever mad reason, of a documentary I saw showing an Asian girl's prearranged marriage. All the females come together before the ceremony to help dress the bride and her body is painted in bright colours of celebration and here I sit, the centre of attention, and my heart races in fear. I back away, standing now looking at my family and friends, an outsider in my own life, and I wonder again have I gone insane. Is my normal life somewhere else for the taking while I live in a closed mind of madness? Just two weeks ago I had pottered in the chemist trying to choose a nice colour to highlight my hair and now today I talk of wigs. What folly has control of my life? Will I be strong enough to cope? Later, alone and frightened, I feel my naked head. I look in the mirror and to my surprise I see a reflection of a new me, strong, brave and full of determination. My will to live is unimaginable.

***

Today it is decided I will venture into town with my Mam and sister Pauline to go wig hunting. For the moment I borrow a scarf belonging to my Mam. Its silky cloth slides on my head and its irritation makes me cranky. Its alien feel is a constant reminder of its necessity. But I suppose today my main worry is, 'Will people stare?'. Mam calls a taxi – I can't face the journey on the bus. I am so vulnerable and weak and already embarrassed at the thought of the assistant in the shop looking at my bald head – and what if there are other customers?

When we arrive at the shop I am relieved to find it quiet. It was a good idea to go mid-week and early morning. The assistants act as though they see bald heads every day, and I suspect they probably do. Not everyone is purchasing for a different look or a fashionable change of style, so I relax as she displays the different options available to me. She casually asks questions about my previous crown and glory, and I kick myself I didn't bring a photo of me before my hair loss. It would have helped greatly with colour, choice and style. The poor girl has nothing to work on, as even my eyebrows and eyelashes have gone now. She brings a variety of choices and explains the different price range.

You learn something new everyday, sometimes things you wish you never had to know. It is explained that I can get an allowance in part payment for my wig from the Health Board. Of course the lower-priced samples are not the ones you would pick by choice and I feel sorry for anyone whose options are restricted by finances at this sensitive time, a time when things should be made as easy as possible. Imagine that finances can hinder you replacing something so personal and treasured! I am extremely fortunate that I can afford to choose and I know in my heart that, even if I couldn't, my family would see me right.

Time passes and I begin to feel nervous as choices begin to run out and nothing seems right for me. My sister has cracked up laughing at a few of the options! We have all seen these wigs at some stage – the dull brown wig that looks like it's made from nylon and bears no likeness to any human head of hair. It is good we can laugh, but I feel it is laughter weighted and tainted with nerves.

I feel bewildered. Wigs are meant for dressing up, for Halloween. I have had one for years. It has spent time at many a party and has been paraded from door to door on a tiny head of trick or treat. It is always retrieved from the attic for times of merriment and fun. How things change, and so fast.

I feel the assistant's patience begin to wane and I feel panic rise inside me. My options flitter away. God, what will I do if I find no wig to suit me? How will I cover my head? I cannot walk the streets looking like Kojak! What about children? They would scream with terror and fright. I feel I would really be shoving my illness in people's faces. I just wish I didn't care. How easy would that be? I stare confused in the large shop mirror. A face reflects, drained, grey and frightened, and I want to run and run to the end of the earth. I want to scream until I am hoarse but instead I look to my Mam and Pauline and announce determinedly, 'Let's go! I can't do this! It's not for me.' And they look relieved and agree, 'No, it's not you!' I am embarrassed that I have wasted so much of the assistant's time but I find the wigs restricting and itchy. And it's pointless – I know in my heart the wig would never see the light of day. We make our excuses and leave. I have used my quota of energy for today. Mam hails a taxi and we head home. Tomorrow is another day. We can always shop for bandannas.

***

The taxi man is friendly and ventures to ask, 'Well ladies, a good day's shopping?' I tense. The question hangs awkward, unanswered, hovering in the air. New territory. My new life. I reply calmly, 'No we were shopping for wigs. I have lost my hair. I am unwell.'

I want to be strong, to face the world head on, to face this illness head on. I will take what is thrown at me. I will not hide. This is all new, a blank page. I am testing the waters of my new life. I receive words of sympathy, words that will accompany me for the coming months. Nearly always these are paper-clipped to a story – a story of some friend's cousin's brother who has cancer – and I find I become detached, unable to listen to the tales of woe. The taxi driver's words are a jumble to my ears. I cannot bear to listen today. Maybe when I am stronger.

This story-telling is one human trait that has made me smile inside since I was diagnosed. I sometimes wonder why people tell you their cancer stories. Is this an Irish thing? Is it a nervous thing? Is it a way to let you know they have some understanding? I find I am conscious of words, of the reaction from people hearing for the first time that I am unwell. Some have a litany of question on my diagnosis – I have learned this usually comes from those with hypochondriac tendencies!

'How did they find out you had cancer?'
'Were you sick for long?'
'Could you see your lumps or just feel them?'
'Where exactly were they?'
'What other symptoms did you have?'

And on and on comes the barrage of questions. 'It must be terrible to lose your hair. Does ALL your hair go, everywhere?' I read these questions on the faces of those around me. Curiosity, a natural human reaction, one that I would have if it were someone I knew. And eventually the question is asked. Sometimes in a natural, concerned conversation that flows without thought between those close to you. Other times it is awkward and stilted, concealed in innuendo. And I respond with one of my many rehearsed answers; I answer with empty words, with no emotion, withholding the reality, the unimaginable loss, the humiliation and the sadness. I explain: 'Well, firstly it depends on the mix of drugs you have to take; some people's hair thins, other's goes all patchy, but I have lost everything and I mean everything.' I see the shock but their curiosity is satisfied. But I know that these are all natural human responses. I understand that mostly people have good reason to be afraid.

Cancer is everywhere, or maybe it just feels like it's everywhere – like when you're pregnant and it seems there are pregnant women everywhere, stalking you. I suppose it is all about awareness and human nature. If something doesn't interest you it can go unnoticed in your private world. I try to remember how I responded when I had been confronted with a person who suffered a serious illness. I was probably guilty of being too straightforward or maybe I fumbled some stupid question with my nerves out of control and then probably beat myself up about it later.

***

Aine Ni Bhrion, a friend, brought me a journal today and wrote inside: 'Janette, this little journal is solely for recording all the positive thoughts that go through your mind each day. PS I will be checking your homework.' I don't know if I can keep it all positive, but I will try. I write words every day and I make myself list positive thoughts. At first they don't just appear; it is an effort. Here is an example:

Good thoughts for today
my hair will grow back
I will get better
I must take each day at a time
my Angels and St Anthony are guiding me
I have the love of Graham, Declan, my
mam and dad, family and friends to keep
me strong

I have to make time in the hospital chaos for myself to acknowledge the good things surrounding me. This is an enormous necessity, but it is not an easy task when there is nowhere to be alone for one minute.

Another day of positive thoughts
A huge amount of people get cured (I am
going to be one of them)
next week will be my second chemo over
One of the worst parts of my chemo is behind
me (hair loss)
more people believe I will be okay*
People are praying for me and thinking
positive thoughts

***

26 February 2001

I return to the hospital for my second lot of chemotherapy. I attend the Day Ward for one session. I am quiet, like an obedient, unquestioning child. 'Hi Janette, we just need to

---

* I decided to send out word that I wanted everyone to really believe I would be well again and if they truly believed it, I felt sure I could be well.

check you in. Can you wait in the secretary's office?' 'Hi Janette, can we just run through your details?' I stare straight ahead, I can't bear to look at the other patients, their thin, pale faces or their bloated, bandanna-covered heads, so I sit silent. 'Janette Byrne. Is Janette Byrne here? Follow me.' The nurse chats happily, 'Hi Janette, how are you today? Cold out there isn't it? Have a seat there. Sorry, can you remove your cardigan? We need to get at your arm.' Declan stays close as though he fears I might die or disappear forever. The doctor comes, 'Hi Janette, can you come over here and lie on this bed please?' I strip to my pants and bra and she gives me a full check from head to toe, a full NCT. I have little will or energy. My arms flop on the bed when she lets them go. I feel lost and confused. I spend the afternoon in the ward getting my chemotherapy; people come and go over and over. God, I never realised so many people had cancer. I wonder how many of us will live. The doctor speaks soft, soothing words as tears run down my face. I don't make a sound, just tears. 'Are you okay Janette?' and I whisper, 'I just don't want to die. I am too young.' She smiles, 'Janette, you'll be fine. You have a great chance. You're too lovely to die. Try not to worry. We will look after you.' I feel no comfort from her words. Already in my heart I know it is too soon to tell. I leave the ward feeling dishevelled and wrecked, as though I have done two-hundred rounds with Barry McGuigan. I head home shattered.

***

When my pals Aine and John arrive to visit me I feel nervous. It is strange to feel this way in the presence of people you have known for years and have always felt relaxed and comfortable with. The lump burning in my throat doesn't help. I want to burst out crying. These are new feelings I experience towards close family or friends on the first encounter since being diagnosed. Somehow I mostly manage to keep it together, smile and pass over the initial awkwardness and tell the story to date.

While John and Aine are visiting, a call is returned from HUG, a cancer support group for Hodgkin's Lymphoma patients. I rang them yesterday wanting to talk to someone who had survived my type of cancer. This need came on like a bolt from the blue, a burning in my soul; this urgency to hear a voice, to hear the words spoken fresh and honest and to know this person still lives a healthy life. I pine for the words, 'I am alive and I had Non-Hodgkin's Lymphoma.' It is a woman on the phone. She was a young girl, just sixteen, when it was discovered she had Non-Hodgkin's Lymphoma and that was around twenty years previous. I speak to her for a short while and am grateful for her call.

That night I lie in bed thinking about her, analysing our conversation and I wake with the alarm rising again. It hadn't worked. I need someone who was my age when they were diagnosed. There has to be more common ground. Words play in my mind, words I have heard somewhere in passing: 'Chemo works much better if you are very young.' These words have made an impact. I let the negative thoughts in, dissolving any chance that I will feel better from her call. I decide I have to speak to someone with exactly the same ailment and around the same age. I lift the phone in urgency and explain my needs.

The next day I speak to a woman in her thirties who has been in remission for three years. Relief floods over me. It comes to me as clear and positive as any notion that has ever entered my head: 'If there was one survivor, well, there would be two.' I resolve that I will be this second survivor; I will be well again; I will live. I write in my diary, 'I will probably have the poor girl tortured with questions.'*

---

* Thank God I never felt the need to speak to her again.

March 2001

16 March 2001

Back in hospital for my third session of chemotherapy – a five-day course – and another operation. I am not due in until 20 March but I have to go in early to hold my bed. The thought of going in really upsets me but I put on a brave face for my family. I have a sleepless night as I am very sick. But I can cope because I know at this journey's end I will be well. During the night I press the panic button, a first for me, but a necessity. I don't think I can make it to the loo alone and I need to vomit. It is dark and still in the ward. But for the heavy breathing of deep sleep, all is quiet. I press the bell again. I am frightened. I feel I am going to pass out, things just don't feel right. I feel the vomit rise and I stumble to the loo, head spinning. No one comes. I am alone and terrified. I leave the door ajar in the hope that someone might see or hear me. The nurse arrives, shocked and concerned. 'Why did you not call us, Janette?' She comforts me while I throw up over and over in the basin. I am glad she is there and I feel safe. I am so weak. Eventually she helps me back to bed and gets me a container and some medication. It is discovered later the panic button was not working. Thank God I was only just calling to be sick.

***

I hate my chemo so much, the smell and those bright colours. I hate the hum of the machine as it times the liquid pumping through my body. I lie awake staring at my 'enemy' as it overtakes my body, indiscriminately killing my cells, good and bad. But I know with the little bit of clarity I have left that I must embrace my treatment and try to understand it. I start to call it my friend, relax a lot more and begin to realise that this is my hope, my hero here to save me in my hour of need. I think of the people who studied for years to gain the knowledge to invent something like chemotherapy and the other drugs I must take and I thank God for them. My heart feels for the people years ago that were given no hope and suffered horrendous pain only to die a slow, miserable death. They were not so fortunate.

I know that the men, women, girls and boys who are being treated the same time as me are all different, but I think fear unites us and the terror of the situation makes me get to know people quicker than I have ever done in my life. It's hard to be someone you're not when you share a room for months with seven strangers; you eat, sleep, puke, cry and maybe even die with these women. Mostly we all just want our lives back; we want to be healthy and happy again. There are so many long hours to kill and lots to talk about. We have so much to worry about that pretences have no place here. The effort that pretences would bring would just be too much extra strain. Most days our emotions are so raw and exposed you can nearly feel the pain in the room, especially those horrible times when someone dies on the ward. It engulfs us and drags us to a place so sad and lonely it takes a lot of support and clarity to return and fight another day.

***

For those of us who can't face the wig shops some ladies visit the hospital ward selling wigs. Their visit brings with it an air of excitement. Some of the girl's parade for us the different options they might choose. We laugh at some – they are just so horrible. They look like someone scraped them off the M50 on a wet day! I can't believe somebody actually makes them and expects a human to wear them. I find I am nervous as some of the girls try the wig options. A straightforward honest person by nature, I fear I will offend if the choice is hideous and I say so. I play it safe and leave the advice to others. I don't want to be part of this scene. I long so much to be shopping for clothes with my pals, not wigs. But mostly I want to be well and free.

***

Invent a solution to end this indignity

I feel a sickness burning in my gut and I battle with its symptoms. At first it seems confined; then I feel its tentacles flick, flick against nerve endings, bristling, sending darts of frustration through my body. I feel irritated and cranky today. Am I looking for a reason, waiting for a simple irritation so I can leap at it and blame it for my frustrated mood? I never want to blame my cancer. I feel that would be fruitless, pointless and debilitating. But this anger is constant, buried, suppressed since the beginning.

I had the same irritation last week as I sat with one of my visitors, a friend from work. A nurse came to my bed, chart in hand, greeted us both and then asked, 'Janette have your bowels moved today?' I respond without a second's delay in a voice devoid of any emotion, a voice mundane and dead, 'Why, did yours?' I just couldn't help myself and I hated myself as the nurse's eyes flew from the chart, mouth open, eyes popped and a sullen realised response, 'Sorry. I will come back later.'

My anger's source today is a measuring jug; a simple, fecky, plastic measuring jug. And my anger … I will explain so you don't think I have totally lost the plot. I perch above the filthy toilet, legs weak and wobbling from my weight, unbalanced with strain and weakness. I clutch my drip stand, misreading its ability to steady me. I try to keep the drip tubes from contact with the toilet as they feed my chemo through my body. And in my other hand a plastic jug, its duty to collect my bladder contents. I hate this procedure. If you are a woman then I am sure you already understand why I struggle. Squatting, as my tummy warns that my bowel also considers emptying its lot. The chemo and antibiotic send our bowels mad, constipation one day, diarrhoea the next. I feel I am never free from the stupid drip and I want to rip its grip from my arm and run from this place to the sea or the mountains, anywhere but here. Yet my shadow remains. His squeaky wheels a constant; his unrelenting tug at my chest or arm also a constant. When I move suddenly he yanks me back to position. He is acting like a wayward shopping trolley today and I am in no mood. But I am sure you have gathered I am no mood for a lot of things today.

What is my real gripe? The plastic jugs of urine lined like soldiers on the toilet window ledge? My drip stand and its relentless presence in my world? I feel the anger start today as I wobble above the loo, urinating on my hand, faeces also a contender and my face burns with anger. I want again to flee this sewerage-smelling, unventilated hole. I return to the ward with a furrowed brow and am heartened to hear I am not alone in my moans. We chatter about how disgusting and awkward we find this practice and how we hate the constant silent companion who never leaves our side. I hate my natural bodily functions now, another thing that was normally unheeded in my previous life but, hey, this is cancer with all its trimmings. I know these trials are part of the bigger picture to save our lives and I should really stop moaning. I have a chance, yes; I am being treated, yes. Others are not so lucky. I am sorry, please forgive me.

***

I have realised something very important today: I am still in shock. It has not left my mind and heart. I lie awake, staring into the night, worrying for my sanity. I feel every thought, and every emotion, has moved to another zone, another dimension. I no longer live in the same world as my family or friends. I have moved to a place where everything is fragile, where things no longer just are, everything is heightened, every thought counts, every action counts. I am terrified, happy, sad, lost, in love with life but mostly I am lonely as I travel this cancer path in solitude as one being. As my treatment continues, week in week out, I hold it together as best I can. I must wait the long wait for the end, whatever that brings. I feel sorry for myself tonight, but I have no right to: some of the girls have already lost the battle but I still have a chance, I still have hope. She is my companion; she keeps me sane. She wraps her arms around me and I sleep at ease for the remaining few night hours.

Sometimes I have daydreams. What if I change my name and move to another country? Why did I not go to London when I was twenty-five when I had given it consideration? Would any of these things have made a difference? Would I have escaped this disease? I know they are crazy thoughts, but consider my mental state! How is my brain coping as my body is constantly pumped with chemotherapy, drugs whose names have become frighteningly familiar to me?

We are lonely souls now. No one can say the right things. No words will soothe our hearts and nervous smiles on the faces of everyone in our life make us feel for them. They are lost also in unfamiliar territory, in an alien world of fear. Yet all the while we try to pretend all is okay. It is a deranged world where I now live, trapped, pleading every minute for my life. Oh, to be one of the fortunate, reprieved with the chance to carry on with the wonderful gift of life.

Awake at night, I look around the dimly lit ward at the other lonely patients, most unrecognisable to friends who have not seen them in a couple of weeks. Hair gone, face pale and bloated, fear glaring from their eyes like cornered animals. We all look frighteningly similar – like a new race of people! All the fluids we must take make us restless and we constantly pass each other through the night back and forward to the toilet. Sometimes while I sit perched on the side of the bed waiting for someone to finish I watch the scene: bald heads, frail, stooped bodies with drips attached, sleepwalking to and fro. It reminds me of a bad horror movie I watched as a child, which kept me awake for weeks wetting the bed with fear.

I have always believed everything happens for a reason but I just can't see any possible reason for all of this to be happening to me. It was as though I hold the end of a kite and a storm carries me further and further out of control, further away from my starting point, from my life. And while I float on the winds the loneliness intensifies. No one can understand how I am feeling, no one.

I try desperately to make some sense of my new life. What did I do wrong? Had I not eaten the right foods? Maybe I had too many late nights and drank too much alcohol when I was younger. Maybe it's the hate I felt for the friend whom I once loved but could not forgive in my heart. Maybe it's a tumour of loathing growing in my chest, wrapping itself around my wind pipe, sucking the air from my lungs. If only I could have forgiven and moved on. Is this my own doing? My mind races round and round. Questions, questions with, it seems, no answers.

God, I am so afraid; nothing is the same. My whole life has been swept from under me. Everything I knew as normal has been taken away. I must try to keep my head together. I have decided this is my most important task if I am to wake from this nightmare. I have realised that these events are beyond my control. So I must accept all that has happened and pass my life over to complete strangers. I must accept. These are the words I say to myself as I lie awake, my mind pulsing with thoughts of doom. Accept your illness. Accept your treatment. Accept your hair loss. Accept the fear and your new way of living – hospital, week after week, day after day, until you no longer feel safe in your own home.

I watch the terror in the faces of my family and friends and know that this time Mam and Dad cannot help. There are no creams hiding in the bathroom cabinet used for years to heal all our ailments. My parents are with me on this journey of terror. What can I do but accept. Someone tell me, is acceptance my only friend? Will it keep me sane as I lie again sweating, staring into the darkness, away from all that is familiar to me? I have the urge sometimes to react like a deflating balloon and go flying uncontrolled through the streets screaming, weeping, roaring at the top of my voice for someone to help, 'Please someone take me away from this nightmare, from the horror that has become my life.' But what good would that do? I still have my cancer. I lie in the ward drained of all will. It is so weird: it's as though every particle of joy has been drained from my body. I have become a zombie – I even look and walk like one. Janette no longer exists.

***

The nurses seem giddy today. One of the girls is getting married soon and her hen party is on this weekend. In the distance I hear their girly chatter and I am comforted by the normality of their lives. It seems only yesterday that this was my liberty also. I hear the giggles as they try to catch the bride-to-be for a daytime bath. I smile and revisit memories of my own life. Their banter gives me a will. I want to be in that place again; I want to be well, to be carefree, stress free. I want life, my life. I feel their fun like a drug soaking into my heart, spurring me on, reminding me that beyond these walls my life is waiting. Now I just have to get well and continue where I stepped out. I think of Lourdes, a Filipino nurse – a gentle, kind lady. I watch the lonely look in her eye when she speaks of her family and her home thousands of miles from here. I admire her strength as she works each day to support their life. Even in the misery of a cancer ward there is inspiration everywhere.

***

A young girl of about eighteen has been brought to the ward today. I feel for her. Apparently they believe she may have diabetes but have stuck her in with us crocks. I see her stare nervously at us. Her mother has somewhere to be and must leave and we hear the girl pleading for her to stay. We all play the usual game of 'let's pretend the curtain is a wall and that we didn't hear a thing'. Her mother is adamant and says she will return soon and then, for whatever reason, she leaves. What a bore for a teenager to be stuck with a gang of oul' ones! She lies still in her bed, listening to her CD and staring at the ceiling. I try a smile but it is not returned.

A young fella arrives now to visit our new patient and it seems the sight of his girlfriend in a bed is more than he can bear. We hide embarrassed behind books and magazines as they slurp and suck, lips locked in teenage passion. It is hysterical. Us adults mortified as the hands roam under the blankets and the breathing increases from both parties. Thank God at this stage a very feisty young nurse comes in. We watch her expression go from a smile of greeting to us all, to confusion as she follows our eyes and, like a grandmother of old, she lets rip: 'Hey you two, give it up! My God, will you stop that carry on? Now come on, that's it! Out with you. Out!' All she was short of doing was grabbing him by the ear.

Both youths had the respect to at least go red and the boy skulked from the ward, his pride bruised. Needless to say the girl never spoke to any of us for the two days she spent on the ward. It was just like a daytime TV drama live in the ward for our entertainment. Oh, to be young and in love!

***

What have I now become? Will I still be here when I have finished my treatment, me as I was before, or have I gone somewhere else, to another place, unable to bear this time? Am I already the new me? Will I be a better person or will I live in anger and frustration, unable to move on and let go? Will my life be tainted, scarred by this intrusion? How can I feel safe knowing that this disease sneaked around my body undetected, working internally to destroy me? Was it there within me when I lay in the sun on holiday or gathered with family celebrating another Christmas warmed in contentment? Or while I lay with my love in a dishevelled bed, was it with us, undetected, devious? Was it always there, waiting until it had infiltrated enough cells, dragging me down lower and lower to a point when all my strength was drained and I was left weak to the vein? How can I ever trust myself or any doctor to know when this thief may be there waiting again to rob me of my life? Can my life ever be the same? Will this treatment work? Will I live? What lies in store for me? Will I die?

***

Lily

'Jesus yer passing me round like snuff at a wake,' said Lily, a very agitated eighty-year-old cancer patient. One thing is clear: Lily has had enough. I envy her. No messing around with Lily, she says what she feels. She whispered to me from behind a wrinkled hand the seriousness of her situation with what seemed to be no emotion: 'The big C, ye know, lungs, from smoking, can't operate, too old.' That was it. Her medical record to date: clear, precise, short and swift. It would take her doctors hours of deliberation to decide prognosis and procedures, but in Lily's mind there was no need for all that carry on. It was the big C and that was that.

They seemed to be having trouble finding a ward for Lily and had apparently moved her four times in less than a week. This to Lily seemed more of a problem than her illness and it was making her very cranky. Now we would all suffer her tiresome moaning about everything, from the blood they were draining constantly from her veins leaving her with nothing, to the fact that they were more interested in drugging her than making her better. But I loved to listen to her challenge them. Lily took no shit. She once asked a very matronly, pain in the ass nurse if she'd ever thought of presenting *The Weakest Link*; she then proceeded to stare out the window as if something of untold interest had attracted her immediate attention, leaving the rest of us on the ward wondering if we had heard her correctly. Later, when asked by our nurse of joy could she move so her bed could be made, she replied, quite sharply and with a look so wicked even Joan Collins would be proud, 'And what if I said no? What then nurse?' God! Such entertainment, and all before 8.00 a.m.!

***

I don't really relish the thought of another operation but I have little choice now that my veins have all but given up and any attempt to access them is causing me huge discomfort. On my next trip to hospital a Portacath* will be fitted, and I will receive five days of chemo. This device will be used every day

---

* Implantable access device inserted surgically under the skin in your chest into a large vein. Size 20–25cm long.

for access instead of my vein. But I worry about the operation. Am I strong enough? Will I die? I push the negative thoughts aside and plant seeds of positivity in my brain. I soothe myself with these words: 'This instrument is a necessity and will bring you great relief. The team are brilliant and they know what they are doing, trust them.' I sit in a wheelchair, waiting. The porter jokes and laughs; one fella whistles and sings, and through a smile he says, 'Don't look so scared. You'll be grand.' And I reply very quickly with a cheeky grin, 'You told me that the last time and I ended up with cancer!' He looks at me in hope of a joke but I am wheeled on, leaving him bewildered. I am such a bitch sometimes!

20 March 2001

I have been in hospital now for three days – not getting chemo, just holding my bed. Three unnecessary days I could have spent with my family. For others who must do the same they are days lost that they will never, ever have the pleasure of again. This has happened a few times to me at this stage. I am still relatively new and still learning about the disastrous Irish Health Service and the juggling that must take place in an overcrowded and chaotic hospital system to accommodate us all. It is frightening for me to know that my consultant is not in control of my access to a hospital bed and my treatment.

I believe the problem for cancer patients is that there is no dedicated cancer ward. I am told also that a serious bed shortage is causing hundreds of people around the country to wait months for operations and treatment. I worry, what if there was a major disaster in the country, a plane crash, a train crash? It happens elsewhere, it could happen here – we are not untouchable. We have in the past had our disasters: I remember the Dublin bombings, the Monaghan bombings. What would happen to those of us with long-term illness in the wake of a disaster? Would we be left at home for months without our treatment? I cannot see how they could cope, as the hospitals cannot cope already with the normal day-to-day demands the population put on our Health Service. These are genuine worries that fill my already worried head. But I try not to think about what may never happen. We no longer have any control of our lives, we are totally dependent and it terrifies me.

26 March 2001

I am glad to be home again after ten days in hospital. Declan and I are staying with my parents again. I try to muster some energy so I join in playing cards with my family. But my heart is not in it and I get out of the game after a short while. I am knackered – even sitting up in the chair is a chore and any concentration I once possessed has left the room.

***

It is freezing cold but I try to take advantage of my good days and today is one. We go for a walk in Blessington Park to feed the ducks, something I love. I never seem to bring enough bread, as I always end up feeding the gulls and magpies, feeling sorry for them in their struggle at in-flight theft. I revel in the sight of the bluebells and snowdrops. I absorb the beautiful vestment purple of the crocus and it warms my heart. I am magnetised towards nature in its innocence and selflessness. Nature is always there, patient, silent to our busy ears. She calls to us but we cannot hear. She is smothered by the roaring traffic. Her birds sing an unheard song. Her breeze whistles a melody through her trees and we are oblivious. Nature stays with us always waiting, free to us to delight in her pleasure but always in our own time. I find a peace in its sight and calm in its embrace. I suck the fresh air into my lungs as though storing it for a later date. It is indescribable the peace in my heart as I escape the hospital confinements. I try to make the most of my few days' break before I must return but first I need peace and quiet and a moment's space to recharge, before I venture home to my worried family, friends and neighbours.

***

I wake up to the phone ringing. My brother Brendan and my sister-in-law Isobel phone to see if I would like to go away with them. They have hired a boat on the Shannon for the weekend. I am surprised by my instant reaction – dread and near panic at the thought of being away from the hospital, away from my carers. Thoughts rush through my brain, 'What if I got a bug? What if I passed out? What if I needed help?' I struggle to find an excuse and feel very guilty. They had extended this caring offer and I was giving fear the permission to stifle any chance of fun and relaxation. Common sense tries a determined voice in my brain: 'Go on, get away and have some fun. You should try to forget about everything for the weekend.' Fear replies for me before I get the chance: 'Yeah sure, like she could do that!' I decline their offer with a sad heart. Fear has won again. I never thought in a million years my days would be ruled by fear.

***

30 March 2001

I'm back in hospital today – I'm neutropenic*. My time at home was way too short, but it was nice to have the time in familiar surroundings. I hate going to hospital. I hate packing

---

* Neutropenia is a haematological disorder characterised by an abnormally low number of white blood cells.

that stupid bag again. I hate my cancer. I bring a jigsaw of a lighthouse to the hospital hoping in some way to keep my mind distracted.

Today I wake and from the onset I feel miserable. I am frightened so Declan calls the nurse for reassurance that all is okay. I have terrible headaches. They are a norm following chemo but sometimes I let imagination and fear play together and the result breaks the wall of sense and understanding that keeps me strong. Today is one of those times and I need to dispel the notions that imagination and fear have planted in my brain. I need to dispense with the trail of negative thoughts they have strewn like Hansel's crumbs, leading me to the path of doubt and thoughts of a brain tumour forming in my head. They have done such a good job I can feel the phantom tumour pound its presence through my skull. It has been explained to me before why these pains rack my body. It is normal after chemo. Your body starts to get weaker and weaker as the chemo depletes good and bad cells. It would take a specialist to explain medically exactly what the chemo is doing inside but for me this is enough information. This phase is called neutropenic, a phase when blood levels drop and God only knows what else is happening. In my mind I know I have a calm understanding of this but some days I am weak. It feels as though my body is screaming from the inside out and I am very aware things are going pretty much haywire inside me: mouth sores, headaches, back pain, weakness like I have never known, chest pain – you name it! I feel a total wreck. This is the hard battle. Every time, I try to keep upbeat and remember that this phase has passed before, but worry seems to linger with me today and I wonder has she nothing else to do.

Lazy bones

I have to mention something that drives me nuts: doctors tying a plastic glove around your arm when they are taking blood. I swear if one more doctor does this I will wrap it round their neck. It really hurts. I wish they would try it on themselves and have the experience of it. It pinches and digs into your arm. For those of you who have never had blood taken and for the doctors who are unaware, there is an item called a 'tourniquet' invented for the purpose of taking blood, but through total laziness most doctors still just use the nearest plastic glove. I urge patients to be strong, please speak out and don't let them hurt you more than is already necessary!

***

A typical day on the ward

We are woken around seven every morning. The routine never changes. Nurses pull the blinds and the windows are opened, regardless of sun, rain or snow. These activities along with the arrival of Dracula (as we humorously call the haematologist) begin each day. Dracula fills her little vials with our blood and already too much is happening for me, a morning slugger. We all wait patiently for the coming hours to find out the results. We have become familiar with the blood levels needed to allow us home for a break and those that will worry us for the days to come. We bug the nurses regularly for any updates on what our blood contents have revealed.

I find this time of day strange in the ward. The early morning brings fresh staff, ready for a busy day and bustling with energy. For us it is quite a lethargic time, as we struggle to come to grips with our surroundings. Most of us sleep poorly; this and the weakness of illness can make it a chore sometimes to even prop ourselves up for breakfast. We smell and hear the arrival of the food before it is in our sight; the mix of toast, porridge, eggs and stewed tea rattles along the corridor on a catering trolley. The odour is enough to turn even the strongest tummy. We all agree that the chemo seems to heighten our sense of smell, reminding those who have had a pregnancy of the early days when someone's perfume could make you retch.

For breakfast I usually choose porridge. I have discovered it is a better option than soggy toast and rock-solid boiled eggs. Some of the girls balk at the sight of the porridge – they can't believe I eat it – but it is something we had always eaten at home as children and in some way it brings comfort. Other mornings, good auld faithful cream crackers and cheese are produced from our private stash and we ignore the hospital fare. We usually eat pretty much in silence. Once we have done the initial check for each others' welfare and have given a helping hand to those who struggle with fiddly jams and butters, we eat our breakfast and usually stare vacantly to the ward, each of us alone and struggling to face another day.

I have always found mornings a drag, but I never thought they could be this bad. I wake now each day to an alien, nightmare world, over and over, again and again, and a dread that never seems to lessen. I find it takes me time each morning to come to terms with what has happened in my life. I start by calming my mind and soul so I can function for another day. Mornings now make me sad. Sad for the loss of my wonderful life, and again I beat myself up for not noticing how every second was spent and for the time I wasted foolishly through my life – days, hours, minutes, seconds, every one of them now seems a treasured gift.

Those well enough now stroll to the shop for morning papers, while others sneak out for a quick fag before the doctor's rounds. Some just take a wander to stretch theirs legs or leave the room to take a breather. We all come back and loll about with lazy sleepy heads. On those days when consultants visit the ward I always sense the nervousness in the air and my tummy turns with anxiety.

The ward is cool and some of us snuggle back under the blankets for a bit of heat. Magazines and papers are read with little interest. The nurses disappear for a shift change and a filling in of our activities during the night. Sometimes the nights have more activity than the days. You never have a dull moment on a ward filled with the waiting. Before my illness I had little trouble sleeping, but in the hospital I battle, tossing and turning. I seem to be always on alert, ears pricked, nervously waiting for something or someone, maybe death. Many a night the nurses kindly bring me hot milk in the hope that it will help me sleep. I always refuse sleeping tablets, but I often wonder if they slip one in on the sly. I really miss my home routine of reading until my eyes close and dozing to sleep in the way of habit. I am deprived this in a communal ward where lights are out at eleven. I hate this routine. But mostly I just hate being deprived the freedom to choose. Hospital is regimental; I accept it must be to work to time schedules, but I miss my freedom so much, just to do what I want to do, when I want to do it. How I had taken this simple gift for granted.

It seems as though breakfast has only finished and dinner arrives: twelve bells. Most days Mam comes in with my dinner. I am so lucky – there is nothing like your mam's homemade dinners. The hospital food can be pretty crap, so on the days when Mam can't bring in my dinner I usually try to manage a sandwich. I feel sorry for the people from the country who don't have this option. We try to make ourselves eat to keep up our strength. I believe it is very important. Over our food and through the day we chat casually about our lives and families, and we bond closer every day. I thank God again for these wonderful women, for the pride and strength they show and the inspiration they are to me.

***

It often strikes me how hard it must be for the patients who are from the country – deprived the necessity of having family and friends close by at this petrifying time of their life. I watch them, lonely and lost with the emotional struggle of cancer. I watch the parents of young girls and boys with cancer juggling long journeys, work and usually other children. I watch it take its toll on the parents as they are forced to shack up in expensive Dublin bed and breakfasts, struggling to stay as long as they can manage, and I watch with a breaking heart the tearful goodbyes as they leave their loved ones behind for another week or so. This horror goes on for months and months, leaving the parents eventually torn to shreds emotionally and physically and, being parents, they deny themselves the luxury of displaying their own feelings for all to see. They veil them well until the battle comes to an end, one way or another. I observe these parents in admiration and I hope I would be so brave and strong if the need ever arose for me.

Can you imagine coming from Kerry to Dublin, months of treatment lying ahead of you, and the phone your only contact now with those you love? And then when you did get a break from treatment you could look forward to a train or car journey for hours. Have you ever had to take a long journey just even feeling a little under the weather? Well, multiply that by a million and you might have some idea how these people feel. I know I find the car journey of twenty minutes home more than I can bear sometimes. We have no idea how these people suffer. You need to be very strong person not to crack. I don't think I would be here without the emotional support and strength I get from my family and friends when they come to visit every day. I can't imagine how it would be if I had to manage week after week alone.

I believe some women opt to have their breast removed rather than put themselves through the ordeal of trips up and down to Dublin for treatment. I suppose that says it all! Are you not ashamed to be Irish when you hear stories like that? I know I am! Ireland, what a country! What a sad place where women make such choices. But, from what I witnessed, who could blame them.

***

My Mam tries to help other patients as best she can. Rose, one of the girls on the ward, lives in Kilkenny and, but for a disabled son, has no other family. Her laundry is causing her great distress as she is confined to bed and is running out of nightdresses and pants. People forget these simple things. I won't get into it but between blood leaks with needles and other accidents you fly through your nightclothes. Mam takes her laundry home and brings them back fresh and clean.* The little help she gives is received with enormous gratitude. Another lady from Cork has us in knots laughing as she washes her granny drawers (as she calls them) and hangs them on the radiator to dry. Well, what option has she? Unless the hospitals can start making arrangements for long-term patient's laundry needs, it still falls on a kind visitor or nurses to help. There is no other option when you are too weak to move, never mind stand over a basin washing your nightclothes and underwear.

***

You might think we have a little luxury. You know at home when you feel miserable, where do you head? Maybe for a nice relaxing shower or a bath, nothing like it to make you feel human or just to get a few minutes of breathing space from others to clear your head? But none of us on the ward

---

* It's only now when we read stories of MRSA and the winter vomiting bug that we realise how dangerous a practice this was.

relish the idea of our daily shower. I will describe for you what it is like. The wait for morning wash or showers begins and with only one shower between six it can be the afternoon before you get a turn. It is a tiny, florescent-lit room. The sani-bin spills onto the floor; some problem not fully explained to us causes a blockage in the sinks creating a disgusting sewerage-like smell. The place stinks, but there are no windows to open! We often joke: maybe they are afraid we might jump. This small area also stores at least two commodes. I hate explaining this but I will. We all get bowel problems and other infections every week from our chemo, so it's necessary to collect a bowel sample to see if we have a bug or if the problem is just a result of the chemo. Well, that is my understanding anyway. Commodes collect our bowel samples and are then pushed into the shower area. We all find this very embarrassing because they could be left for a while if the nurses were busy. And with no window to open … well, I will leave it to your imagination. So when we go for a shower that is our first greeting: the stench of our illness. There's no escaping it; it consumes your nostrils, turns your stomach and is so bad that it occasionally makes me vomit.

Now to the actual shower itself. There is a plastic shower curtain that clings like a static jumper to our skin; its clammy, sticky touch makes me cringe with disgust. We cannot complain about the power of the water from the shower – I often wonder how the tiles manage to stay stuck to the wall. So you can imagine with this flimsy, plastic curtain and battering water, no matter what we do water spills everywhere. The other girls on the ward come banging as the water flows under the door into the ward. And just one final indignity to top it all: there is this huge window (that doesn't open) with no blinds or curtains, and we have to step out of the shower in front of it, displaying for all other windows in the building our full, unprotected nakedness. You have to grapple around for your towel, as there are no hooks and leaving it on the ground means it will be saturated. Now don't forget – we have cancer; we are weak and most of us have gone through recent operations. We are bald. We are vulnerable, but most of all upset, humiliated and fragile.

If I sound like a moan, forgive me, but I need you to know how we suffer apart from our cancer. We could all be dead soon with no one left to tell our story, and I do believe this is why the torture and unhygienic conditions continue. The years and years of fear and silence have left us with this filth. My sister Irene writes letters to everyone who should care. But why should they listen? This is mainly a passing-through ward and most of the families are too distraught to do anything while they are going through the turmoil. When it is over, they either run from the place, joy bursting in their hearts, or crawl away dishevelled and broken, never wanting to set foot there again or hear its name spoken and, I ask you, who could blame them?

April 2001

10 April 2001

After eleven days in the hospital I return to my own home. I need to be in my own home; I need normality. I wake with the sun raying through the curtain gap. Declan stirs from the bed and I roll over consuming all the warm space he leaves in his wake. I lie there pondering, rubbing my hand back and forward on my bald head. Tears sting my eyes as thoughts turn solemn. Many old men are baldy and skinheads choose to be bald, but I feel ugly, unfeminine and frightened. I suddenly realise that the shower has been running now for ten minutes at least and I am instantly angered by Declan's selfishness. This is an age-old argument between us. Declan and his half-hour showers, usually leaving me enough water to wash my big toe.

I jump from the bed and knock on the toilet door shouting, 'Hello, Declan, can you leave me some water?'

The usual response, 'There's plenty, will you stop worrying. I am nearly finished.'

I respond, my irritation trebled, 'Yeah, like every other morning. Jesus, what are doing? You're not that bloody big! Don't be so mean!'

I can't stop – I have to get make my point, 'Look Declan I am not lying. I always run out of water, it's not fair! Why should you have a piping hot shower and I have to do with the dregs?'

I stomp back to bed and dive under the covers like a stroppy teenager. I want to kill him. I mean bash the door down, drag him out and kill him. Anger burns through me. I mutter in my head, 'Selfish pig'. I hear him now turning off the shower. Now the sink taps flow, as he scrubs his teeth, water flowing freely down the sink and I feel I could actually punch a hole through the wall and throttle him. I hear the key turning in the bathroom door and he strolls in like Lord Muck, as only Declan can. Towel tied round his waist, jocks dangling from his hand, he lobs them on the floor. Jesus, he is pushing it. I watch his face, smug and indifferent. The sight of him is like paraffin to a flame. 'It's free,' he says. I glare, 'You don't say.' I take a deep breath and leave the room, still cursing him in my brain, I wipe the steam-covered mirror and see my red, angered face.

I feel funny, angry, irritated. How can we argue when I might die? How can we not when we are normal? And somewhere in my twisted brain I smile, because I'm kind of glad that there is still this normality in my world that has changed now beyond recognition.

***

This morning I am alone in the house. Making toast for my breakfast I set the grill ablaze. Normally I would be clear thinking, take control and sort it out. But today I am panicked and run to the street, calling to a man passing, a complete stranger, 'Help me, please, my cooker is on fire.' He runs to the stove, slowly pulls out the tray and covers it with a damp cloth. Calm and collect, no panic, just like I used to be. And here I stand watching, like a blundering idiot, shaking from head to toe. I am not safe to be left alone. I am normally strong and independent but it seems now that it's not just my appearance that is changing, and this upsets me greatly. I was never a girly girl and now here I am, this panicked damsel in distress, running to the street dragging strange men to my home. He could rape or murder me, whatever, but I don't think I would really care. I don't know what worries me most – the panic, the silliness, maybe it all. When my hero leaves I sit in the chair and cry tears of frustration, tears of loss and fear. I find this new me has begun to evolve nervous and weak. If someone drops something or bangs a door I jump ten feet off the ground. I feel I am changing every day, slipping all the time further away from myself.

***

Most days now when I am at home from hospital I stay alone by choice. My family are always near and pop in and out or phone regularly to check on my well-being. I prefer to be in my own bed and my own home. It is normal and I need normal. I decide today to go on the internet and see what this Non-Hodgkin's Lymphoma is all about. I feel like a sneak. Declan has asked me not to do this. His argument is that it will frighten me, but I don't feel I could be anymore frightened. I find all sorts of sites and I read a couple of lines from a few. Declan is right; there is too much information, too many variations. I could end up reading something that really doesn't relate to my grade or stage of Non-Hodgkin's Lymphoma and if I take it all on board I could convince myself I have no hope. The only good outcome is I find a letter from a man in America who had a bone-marrow transplant three years previous and he is still in remission from Non-Hodgkin's Lymphoma. I feel a bit lifted by that, but then I remind myself that you don't know who is putting the information on the internet for us to read – it could be anyone. And even if they are legitimate, I remember that everyone is different. It is very important through your treatment to remember that we are individuals and that the treatment works different on everyone. You also have to take into consideration how someone is feeling in their head. I really believe this plays a huge part in helping us make it through our cancer. If you can keep it together and try being positive, I firmly believe you improve your chances. There was one man in the hospital who was diagnosed with throat cancer. He was a lonely person with no family. He decided the day he was diagnosed he would die. He hit the drink and smoked himself to death. He just had no will. He died without a fight and it made me angry for the waste of his life. I know I have a lot going for me – great family, close friends and a strong will – but some days when things are bad and I am very ill I feel my strength abate and my will slip and I see the path of death lie straight before me, waiting for me to tread alone.

**

Relationships suffer

The three of us lie together in our bed: me, Declan and cancer. The intruder is always with us now even in our place of private retreat. It makes us awkward with each other, that and the little time we share alone, as my time is now divided between hospital and my parents. Visits of family and friends are all very welcome and needed but it leaves little free time for two people to find each other in a maze of complication. Sex, a private time of love and togetherness, is now shadowed by fear and worry. Intimacy stifled, paused in this world of stress. Desire now only a word used in sentences of health and well-being. We lie together holding hands. I need some form of physical contact, some expression of tenderness. I feel so lonely.

**

I have found when I am home for a few days after a session of chemotherapy my heart is breaking for my family. They are lost and try to act normal, to be around me yet give me the space I need. They visit the hospital every day when I am there. When I am at home my friends circle around me and I feel guilty, as though I have dumped my family. I hate this extra burden of guilt and really wish I didn't care, but I would hate to hurt my family when all they are guilty of is caring for me.

***

With the help of wonderful people in my life, sometimes I can forget I am ill. Today was one of those days. It was Easter Sunday and although there was a chill in the breeze the sun shone brightly for our pleasure. I went for a walk on Killiney beach with my family. It was great to just be free of the hospital, to be natural and to be in the fresh, open air, feeling safe and loved. We built castles in the sand and I was relaxed and content. My mind took a break from 'What ifs?'. The seconds were not stained by thoughts of doom and I did not allow disquiet to rape my mind and smother these precious hours with worry and stress. I can see my brother-in-law reading this in the future (a no-nonsense type) and I smile, thinking what he might say: 'It was only a day on the beach like any other. What's the big deal?' For me it was a rare day where my mind was calm and free, and I had fun, something that no longer came easy. I am reminded again of a thought that sometimes passes my mind following days like today: 'If memories go with you when you die then I will be happy and at peace for all eternity.'

A family helpless

I mentioned the other night to one of my brothers, 'I need space in my head from this hospital. I am going mad with the TV roaring.' And the next day a brand new portable CD player was produced. Another night I mentioned in passing how much I felt the cold without my hair and like magic I received a cowl, something procured on one of my other brother's trips to China or Tibet, or he probably contacted some Eskimo family and asked them to send whatever they wore on the coldest day of their year.

I am queried regularly for my needs – food, books; my sisters and mother bring me a vast choice of pyjamas and any toiletries I desire. I only have to utter a word and the item materialises and I have no choice. I let them. I see their pain, their loss, not knowing what to do, how to help, worried I will go and they will never see me again.

They are lost too and the only way they can help is by their support and love. I know I would be the same if it were any of them. Declan's family are the same – flowers, goodies. If only they could all buy my health, without a doubt I know I would be well in one second. Visiting times continue to end with the same lines, 'Is there anything you need?' 'Can we get you anything at all?' I would love to joke, 'Yes, I want new glands, ones that are cancer free.' But we would all cry, knowing that with all the money in the world there is nothing they can buy to change that; nothing purchased in a shopping centre can rid me of my cancer. I am so touched by their care, by their love.

It is not everyone who gets the opportunity to need their family so much. This is a huge test for my family, a test of love and strength and we are surviving. We are a family with a lot of love for each other but we're not big on physical expression; for me it is always awkward when I want to embrace one of my siblings – it is a fumble, a stilted gesture of uncertainty.

***

As I write my thoughts I must constantly remind myself that it is my mind, my head, my thoughts. Maybe no one will relate to these feelings and maybe they will wonder had I been insane through my treatment looking at life this way. But through this illness I have felt such loneliness and sadness, laughter and tears kept me sane. It seems strange to say I was lonely when I was surrounded by people constantly, but no one was ever truly with me. Sometimes I wanted to be alone, to have space away from everyone, away from the sadness reflecting in their eyes, away from the smothering of love. I feel guilty complaining about feeling smothered when I know there are people who have had no support from family and had to depend solely on support groups. I do believe in my heart that the support of my family and friends and their belief that I could be well is one of the reasons I am here today. These were just moments, times that I needed to try to clear my mind, to reconnect with myself, to find out who I was, this new me.

> *A day to remember*
> *As I struggle with my diary and listing positive thoughts, things change.*
> *Today started as a bad day. I didn't sleep last night. I was vomiting and I was frightened and weak. I had my third chemo and was feeling crap. And then I got the results of my bone marrow test. It's clear. Graham and Declan were both with me as I cried with relief. God this is the best news in the world today. Thank you God! I just won the lotto.*

***

It is a fresh Wednesday morning and my friend Christine comes with me to Arc House, a cancer support centre. A 'just to see' trip. We buzz the door and to our total surprise the wall speaks, 'Yes? Can I help you?' What a strange way to greet us? I think if I had been alone I would have run. We giggle in shock and I babble, 'Hello. Eh, can we come in?' Later that day, we laugh about this, conjuring replies we could have spoken on the busy Dublin street as people passed us by: 'Yes, hello. I have cancer and feel like topping myself today. Can I come in?' Or just wailing sobs as people stare at you in horror, petrified to come near you in case they would get involved in something needing their precious time and energy.

My first visit is just to see what it's like. That's it! I am putting out feelers. I mean, counselling is for Americans, who we hear consult their shrinks about what to wear on a night out or what to feed the kids for lunch. I don't really want to get involved in any queer mumbo jumbo and am being very cautious. I flick through pamphlets: 'Living with Cancer', 'Breast Cancer', 'Lung Cancer', you name it – rows and rows of books with horrible words written on their covers. I hate the sight of them. I want covers of happy thoughts – feel-good reading. Books such as *What to do this Summer for that Holiday of a Lifetime, Read this and have Free Shoes for Life* or *Learn to Tango in Ten Easy Lessons.* I want anything but these books for sick people, full of words that are loaded in my mind with sorrow and upheaval. I slyly scan the room. I have to admit the place has a calm homely sense; it is warm and cosy, like a welcomed, loving hug. I look around at others lost in thought and wonder are they also in the alien world where my mind now lives.

A woman comes to talk to us and asks me to fill out a form. This is another annoyance for me. This had also happened when I rang the Irish Cancer Society: What's your name? Where do you live? How many children have you? It all makes me feel like I will soon be a statistic when the weekly cancer patients' details are ready and transferred to the main computer, used I imagine to compile some list for the living of the tragedy that lurks around them. A seed planted in their mind, later to stir guiltily when some buckets shake in their face, a collection for cancer. I want to run or scream, 'None of it matters! I might not be here next month, so can you cut the crap and tell me, Why am I here? Why did I come? And most of all, Why am I so bloody angry?' I fill in the form with a bad heart and sit whispering as though I am in a library, not knowing anymore what I really feel. A gentle voice asks would I like to talk to someone. My heart says no but my mouth betrays me and says, 'Yes'.

I am taken downstairs to a basement office. A smiling face greets me and I relay details as if I am here representing a friend who has temporarily lost her voice. I tell of her ailment; who her doctor is; dates, times. I act well on her behalf and I leave feeling, I don't know, like I just did a good interview. But a thought remains: I have a place to come for whatever lies ahead and I know at least there will be stacks of information should I need it.

***

DAY ONE

17 April 2001: Due in today for fourth session of chemotherapy for a five-day course

What is worse than being told you have cancer? For me it's being told you have cancer, rapid-growing tumours in your chest and being given words of hope; hope and options and possibly a chance to live – 'We don't really know what will be the outcome at this stage, Janette, but we can treat you with chemotherapy and hope it will work' – and then for that hope of life to be snatched away in a sentence: 'Sorry, Janette. We don't have a bed. Try again later.'

Can you imagine the scenario? Me trying my best to be positive, working so hard, focusing on an end, a time span embedded in my brain and a date my goal, and a wait whose end will reveal my fate. How can I get my treatment if there are no beds? My brain seems unable to make sense of what is happening.

I have built myself up so much to be positive and then whack, with one voice, one call, I start to crumble. Negativity finds an opening, a sneaky gap and a split in my wall of strength. He grows, one day, two days, and then the demons speak in my head: 'What is the point in the last two sessions of chemotherapy? It is a schedule, a course, an intensive assault of drugs on your whole system to kill this disease.' I can't help thinking he's right – those treatments are probably wasted now. What is the point? What can I do?

DAY TWO

I sit alone today thinking bad thoughts of death and gloom and he comes loud and strong like a storm in my head. Anger, he shouts to my brain and leaves me fretting like a baby. 'You're stupid. If you sit there and do nothing you will die.' 'I will not die,' I answer him with terror. I shake him from my mind and with resolve I pull myself together. I perk up and from somewhere deep inside I find the will to keep going. I feel this time I have just escaped the black hole of depression, but only by a hair's breadth.

I call Bed Management again: 'Hi! It's Janette Byrne here. I was due in yesterday for my chemo. Is there a bed for me today?' A bored reply: 'Hang on, I'll just check … No, sorry, you will have to call again tomorrow.' I hang up, frustrated and scared, smothering with fear. I can imagine the tumours growing larger and larger, and I let myself cry with worry. I try to accept that this is my fate, that yet again I have no control. What was the point of all my treatment so far? I am frail and weary. I speak to other patients who are further along in their treatment and I soon find out it has been the same for most of them at different stages. They too have played the waiting game. At least I am not fear's only recipient – he has other patients to visit.

One of the other girls who has cancer and is also due back in has become so ill she has ended up in Accident and Emergency on a trolley. I feel so sorry for her and can imagine how terrified she must be. It's a frightening place and, ironically, certainly not somewhere you want to be if you are unwell. I pray that I will be spared that horror. I feel that would surely break any lasting spirit I possess.

What chance do we have? What did we do wrong to deserve this? We don't need this extra torture battering at our minds. I can't believe it. I have worked since I was fifteen and paid all my dues and now the first time I really need this Health Service it is failing me. How can this be? We all pass the hospitals in this country every day, always grateful we look from the outside in and we assume they will be there if we need them, that we will be welcomed into the bosom of safety and healing without hindrance or debate. I try to make sense of the shock I feel to discover that this is definitely not the case.

DAY THREE

I wake again frustrated, my sleep tormented by dreams of doom. I phone Bed Management with a cranky voice:

'Hi, Janette Byrne here. Is there a bed today?'

And the same repetitive reply: 'Janette, sorry, still no bed. The doctors haven't finished their rounds. We won't know until later if there will be one free. So I think it is best if you call back.'

I feel if I hadn't already lost my hair I would defiantly pull it out. I respond losing patience: 'This is stupid. I was due in three days ago for my chemo. Isn't there anything you can do?'

An exasperated voice responds, 'I am just passing on information. There are a lot of other people waiting. You are on the list, sorry.'

'And how many patients are on this list,' I ask surprised and angered.

'About thirty, but you are a priority, Janette.'

And I reply sarcastically, 'Yes, right. Thanks a lot. Goodbye.'

I sit seething with anger and I can't help thinking, 'I bet if it were her sister or mother she would organise a bed pretty quick.' I decide I can try that too – I know someone who works in administration. It's time to call in a favour. Alas, how wrong I am. It appears things are so chronic that no beds means no room at the inn for anyone. And guilt racks my mind. What right had I anyway to try to jump the queue? I battle now with fear and guilt. I don't like being this angry, desperate person. I just want my old life back. I hate this fear.

DAY FOUR

I sleep fitfully and wake disheartened. Part of me wants to rush to the phone but my heart can't bear to hear those negative words again. Today Declan makes the call for me. Still no bed! Friends and family ring every day now to see if I am still here. I feel like an overdue pregnant mam. I try to sound calm in reply to their concern but inside I am terrified. We spend our days phoning and writing letters to TDs, the Department of Health, the Ombudsman – anyone who is anyone. We are just trying to highlight what is happening to me and other patients. We want everyone to know. At least I feel I am doing something and it keeps my mind active, barring at least some of the negative thoughts infiltrating.

DAY FIVE

I sleep little, shaking awake every few minutes, torture spinning round and round in my mind. In the morning it seems as though I awake already crying. I am weary from the fight to beat cancer, to beat the system and I don't know how much more I can take. I hide myself and my tears in the bathroom. My family are stressed enough. I am sure sometimes they wish I were a quiet, more accepting person, but I feel if that were the case now I would surely die. I am glad I am a fighter. The phone seems to ring all day. My Mam is nearly always first to call, her voice dense with concern: 'Any word?' And the words I hate, I speak them like a zombie, 'No. Still no bed.' I know her pain and worry and I feel for her, a mother concerned and stressed. It is so hard to have no options.

DAY SIX

I phone the ward again airing my concerns for the lack of treatment to a considerate nurse. She informs me she will speak to my doctor and ring me back. She returns with the words of someone who cannot help, but genuinely cares: 'We will get you in as soon as possible and Janette, try not to be worrying.' I wish I could take her advice but I have neither the skills nor the serenity not to worry; that is a practice I have yet to learn. I don't feel so good today. I find the weakness the worst. It upsets me and I fight it constantly. I sit writing more letters, making more calls and all the while depressing thoughts leap to the forefront of my mind obscuring everything else. Thoughts of time wasted, vital hours slipping away. And then Negativity clouds my mind with his words of doom: 'Maybe they have realised they can't treat you! Maybe the chemo is not working and they are planning to tell you.' Panic rises in my heart. I try to control the fear. I distract myself again with my calls of desperation.

DAY SEVEN

This has been the longest week of my life. Words repeat over and over in my tortured mind: RAPID-GROWING TUMOURS, HIGH-GRADE LYMPHOMA, RAPID-GROWING CANCER, STAGE TWO, LARGE MASS IN YOUR CHEST. The kaleidoscope of words spins round and round until I can take no more and I snap, and Declan consoles me as I sob like a baby: 'I can't take it. I don't want to die. I want to live. I am so afraid.'

DAY EIGHT

I wake today in a weird, indifferent mood. I feel lost. I feel a bit reckless, giddy, like I don't care if I never went back to the hospital. I don't really let myself ponder the implications of my thoughts. I suppose today I have resigned myself to the pathetic system. Declan phones the hospital. I listen, watching his face for signs. He ends the call, 'Okay thanks. We will call again tomorrow, bye.' I see the sadness in his eyes. I can't care today. I have no will. I turn from him and distract myself.

DAY NINE

I struggle from the bed. The phone is ringing. Three calls, one after the other. Two are from government representatives calling to acknowledge the letters sent by my family and friends to highlight my plight. They sympathise and I listen politely to their political bull and I want to scream, 'All the sympathy in the world won't make me well!' I am untouched by their words. Today I am indifferent, hard. I want to tell them all to shut up and go away and leave me alone.

26 April 2001

I phone the hospital: 'Hi, Janette Byrne here. I am just ringing to see if you have a bed for me.' I wait while she checks and I can't help wondering if these girls hate us or feel sorry for us as we phone them day in day out. She returns uttering words filled with relief, knowing as she speaks them it will stop my repetitive intrusion in her working day: 'Yes, Janette, can you come in as soon as possible. We have a bed for you on St Vincent's ward.' I hang up feeling … I don't know, how do I feel? Relieved, yet miserable that I must go back at all. Elated that I can get my treatment, yet sad because I will miss my family. Happy that I will be safe inside the hospital, but angry that I went through this torture, and so on and so on. For the day my emotions shift in extremes. And so I pack my bag. I hate that bag so much. Once it was packed for breaks away with excitement and joy; now I fill it with dread and fear. I will burn the bag when this nightmare is over.

***

Political games

I am really distressed today. I was prepared for everything, or at least I thought I was. However, it appears politicians have started to use me as a pawn in a war of votes. The Minister for Health Michael Martin has reported I was offered a bed and refused it. I cannot believe his lies. I cannot believe he would think I could be that stupid. I contact the Minister's office and attempt to clear up this untruth. But he is clever. He has tarnished my fight, made people think I am fussy, a liar, and once words have been spoken they are gone forever. He is a very clever man.

Today I receive a letter of apology from the Minister. It appears he was misled by incorrect information. His letter of apology, a sheet of mundane, repetitive words and he without a clue of the upset he has caused me and my family.

Here is a shortened version of the Minster for Health's reply when asked 'to correct the records of the Dail and to explain how this error was made in the first instance'. He basically states that he misinformed the Dail as he was misinformed by the Eastern Regional Health Authority, who in turn say they were misinformed by the Patients' Services at the Mater Hospital. Does any of this seem farcical to you? Does it not send shivers down your spine that these are the people we put our total trust in, our faith in to run our Health Service?

'As previously stated in the house, I am most concerned at the deferral of chemotherapy treatment at the Mater hospital. The patient in question was regrettably unable to be admitted to the Mater Hospital for Chemotherapy on the 17th April due to capacity problems and was subsequently admitted on the 26th of April. This is unacceptable and obviously a cause for great concern to the patient and to myself.'

He has no idea! What can I say? I accept again that this thing is so much bigger than me. I am a minnow in a pond with sharks and I swim on. What option do I have?

Only two of the papers run a tiny article: 'MINISTER IN CANCER APOLOGY'. It boggles my mind why more is not made of his retraction.

***

I have heard that in some country in this mad world they punish their thieves by taking them from prison, bringing them to the town square to have their hand or hands removed in public, only to decide, 'Ah no. We won't do it today. We will leave it until next week.' Over and over this torture continues and eventually the thief would be taken, I imagine totally insane at the final stage, and their hand would be removed. I feel like the thief.

***

Patricia

The ward is eerie today. A new patient is admitted; she is very upset and distressed. She is restless and her mood seems to unease us all. I hear her cry behind a pulled curtain and I walk from the ward to tell the nurse. Time passes but no one comes. A few of us converse with our eyes and hand gestures and I am elected to do the talking. I venture cautiously. What if she thinks we are being nosy or mistakes our genuine concern for irritation at her tears? Patricia is distraught. Mainly because she feels she has no hope, but no one has clarified it for her either way. She is confused and devastated. She wants answers to unasked questions. They remain unspoken, spinning in her head but she dares not utter them for fear they will stir the end. They have told her treatment is not an option, as her cancer has destroyed her lungs. I comfort her as best I can with pretence at knowledge: 'Patricia, you are in the hospital, not a hospice. They must have some hope. You look strong and they are still giving you medication. Patricia there is hope as long as you talk and breathe. Try to be strong.' I am out of my depth, but she seems to calm and I leave her side.

A man comes and wheels her out for a smoke. I cringe at the thought, but what does it matter. It can't possibly make a difference. Lights out and goodnights said but again we hear her muffled cries of distress. Someone presses the bell and a nurse comes. Things settle, but not for long. Patricia begins to ramble and shout into the night. Someone calls the nurse again as Liz, a heart patient, has started to cry and is getting very distressed. The nurse comes and gives Liz some medication. I am so terrified myself. We all feel so vulnerable lying in our beds, weak, ill and exhausted, yet afraid to sleep in case we are woken in fright.

Patricia appears now to be very heavily drugged or maybe the cancer has crept further than she knew. She keeps getting out of her bed. Over and over through the night she struggles with her demons. On the first few occasions the stronger patients in the ward put Patricia back to bed. Time and time again we ring the bell, tormenting the nurse as they tend other very sick patients. I am sure they cursed her and us that night.

Patricia begins pulling her drip from her arm, all the while shouting to us through the night, believing in her demented mind that we are her husband and children. She settles for a while when we remind her who we are and where she is. Then quietness falls and peace nearly manages to take control. The phone rings at the nurses' station. Patricia tries to get to it. She believes it will be her daughter phoning to say she will be late. Peace makes another attempt; exhaustion has arrived. I listen to the unison of laboured breathing but one by one we calm our beating hearts and relax.

Perspiration trickles down my back. I close my eyes, praying over and over for calm. Just as I start to doze I feel a tug at my blanket. In the darkness a skeleton silhouette stands above me, staring vacant and lost. I hold my covers firm as Patricia tries desperately to clamber into my bed beside me. I nearly scream with terror but manage to break through to Patricia's mind and bring her back once again to her nightmare of a life. I give up on sleep and stare vacantly into the night, willing God to bring an early sunrise, a time I hope where everything might seem clearer and calm, might once again be mine. I don't think anyone slept that night. But the saddest thing of all was a nurse apologising to us on Patricia's request the next day. Somehow Patricia had a memory of frightening us and was embarrassed and ashamed. I felt so sorry for her. Two days later we say our goodbyes to Patricia. A hospice space had been found.

***

The world's loss

I don't really want to tell the stories of the deaths, but I would not be true to myself or those lost to us forever if I didn't. Those who are no longer here in body but I know for certain live on in the hearts of those who loved them. My first experience of death in the hospital was of a man in the ward opposite ours. He roared constantly through the day and night, shouting about how much pain he was in. I remember one of the nurses saying, 'That nonsense has got to stop', and that he was just over-acting. He died the next day. I am sure the nurse really regretted her harsh words. His family came through the night to see him, but well before they were notified, we knew he would leave here. Things changed, a mood descended upon us. The word spread around in whispers. Someone took a turn. We all knew he was very bad. He never left his bed or got treatment. Now he has passed on. His daughter arrived. She screamed and screamed, 'That's my Dad. Someone help. My Dad is dead. I want my Daddy.' We all cried, of course, and curled under our sheets like snails retreating into their shells, wondering what way our own family would react if it was us. I will never forget that girl's grief; being lucky to still have a wonderful father alive I can only imagine how she was suffering.

The next death experience for me was much worse: it was one of the girls on our ward. It was a total shock. I remember thinking later that some of the other women on the ward seemed much worse than Eithne. But maybe she was just all out of fight and no longer had the will. I suppose we will never know. She just fell asleep sitting in a chair while we chatted around her, oblivious to her departure. She just never woke up. As far as the staff were concerned it was all very orderly and the death plan obviously came into action. Our curtains were pulled, just to isolate us some more and leave us alone in our terror. The priest arrived. We prayed, mumbling together, numb to the meaning of the words we uttered. The priest and family left and then the person was removed, the zip of the death bag a final goodbye. We lay there, our minds racing, body shaking with fear, too afraid to vocalise what we were thinking: 'Will I be next?' Would it be selfish to say that at the time that person's life ended my main concern was only for me? In all of two hours someone had lived, died, been grieved for and been removed. The bed was remade and everything was supposed to be normal again. And if not that night then the next morning a new patient arrived and, like conspirators, we acted as if nothing ever happened; that Eithne never existed in our world and, of course, the ward routine never misses a beat. It felt so surreal and I wondered the next day if I had in fact dreamt it. Unfortunately for Eithne, it was no dream.

I used to wonder how many deathbeds I had slept in but after my first death experience I no longer cared – it was just not important to me. I remember the way we all acted towards the new patient. It was strange – no one seemed to have the will to talk. We were drained from lack of sleep and fear. We made petty conversation until a day passed and we got the strength from each other to know that everyone is different and it might never happen to us.

It still upsets me to think about the deaths of others so wonderful, so full of life, still capable of laughter and fun even when they knew there was no hope. They held it together most of the time. But we are only human and sometimes the strain became too much and when all visitors were gone the tears would flow. Sometimes a few would cry. I believe we all tried to save our family and friends and each other the tears but sometimes it was as though we had no control. It was as though our tears flowed like a bodily function, a necessity, without emotion.

***

Has this country gone insane?!

There is strange air of excitement about today, the kind of excitement that descends upon a class at end of term or in the office after a hard week on a giddy Friday afternoon. I question one of the other girls if she knows what is going on. Her reply brings a weight of anger and disgust to my heart.

She has heard An Taoiseach will grace the hospital with his presence. I hear some staff and visitors talk about his visit. Their words are a ramble of excitement. I wonder in amazement at my fellow Irishmen and women. I can make no sense of this mood. I would have thought he would be blanked, an unwanted visitor, an undesirable. Yet these people are grovelling and pandering to his call. If I was in control I would deny his entry. I would hang a banner from the roof and scream words of anger at a government who seem indifferent to our plight and a leader who has let the torture of patients continue for years and years. How can he show his face here? I want to fly down the stairs and ruin his day. I want to show him our ward. I want to drag him to Accident and Emergency and I want him to sleep there. I want to tell him how the patients and staff suffer. But sadly I resolve that this man already knows. He just chooses to ignore our plight.

I visualise the scenario: Bertie and his bodyguards surrounded by deluded lick arses. I can see their false smiles, hear their painfully pretentious laughter resounding through the desolate walls and it pains my ears as I stand there alone in my nightgown and slippers, face pale and bloated, shivering in a cold hospital corridor, bandanna covering my nakedness. I muster every last pulse of energy and shout one sentence, a sentence loud enough to be heard above the cackle of deception. One sentence of pride and dignity and they would know instantly all was not well. Stomachs would turn in sickened fear. I can imagine the tut-tuts at the woman who tried to ruin a great day. A murmur would swarm through the crowd and a hustle of strength would drag me from my spot and hide me somewhere to calm my demented mind. But instead, I sit by my bed playing with my imagination and willing myself to go. Go before it is too late. Go have your say. But I sit condemning myself for the fear that consumes my heart and fixes me rigid in my chair.

May 2001

2 May 2001

I decide I need some support from outside my circle of family and friends. I feel stifled. I need space in my head, space for me alone. I decide to partake in one of the relaxation classes in Arc House. This is something I did years ago but could never really get into it. I really must be losing it. You see, me and meditation do not go very well together. My problems are firstly I am a fidget, secondly I am very curious and afraid to keep my eyes closed in case I miss something, but mostly my mind is packed to capacity and wanders at will. I will let you visit inside my head for thirty seconds:

> God. I have to get that price list done for Steven in the Lord mayor's Bar. Ah. look at that poor dog in the street. He looks lost. maybe I should try to catch him. I really will have to do some volunteer work at an animal shelter. I wonder is someone in China really having chicken balls for dinner. why do people let their dogs lick their faces when they obviously know they use the same instrument to wash their privates? Are there really aliens?

So can you imagine trying to lasso my brain, tie it down for one second and begin to clean the slate? I don't think so!

I arrive early for my first class and meet the other people. It is the usual mix of one brave man to five women. We chat, natural chat about the weather and Arc and traffic, and all the while we sit there with our invisible companion, cancer. I find the scene mad. We might all be gone next month and yet we still act so normal. I joke about missing your hair for a bit of warmth and know these words will decide who will like me or who won't. I suppose I will have frightened some with my straightforwardness and they will avoid me. But to my surprise the rules have changed; everyone seems to enjoy the comment and I relax. The ice is broken for me at least and I know I will enjoy these strangers' company.

We settle in the class. The room fills with the scent of geranium oil; it draws me to it, crawling into my mind, whirling around, soothing my inner senses. We lie on the most unusual chairs. They are shaped to your body and low to the ground. Every week someone either can't get in or can't get out and it makes us laugh. We need laughter more than ever. The chairs are so comfortable and along with the warm Donegal tweed blankets we snuggle down like contented babies in a crèche. It seems Mary our instructor has only begun to speak and explain what we will be doing when someone has dozed off. I admire this ability to relax with strangers and sleep. I am disgusted with myself to admit I would care too much what people thought: What if I drooled? Worse, what if I snored, mouth opened wide, snorting like a pig? I could never show my bald head here again, that's for sure! Mary explains the relaxation technique she uses and we begin. I am lucky: without realising it I have secured the window chair and the winter sun singles me out for its rays of heat and well-being. I know now, more than ever, that I need peace of mind and I really want time-out in my head. I close my eyes and listen; the sun, my aide, as I drift to a place of peace and tranquility and I am safe but mainly free of worry. I wander through fields of spring daffodils and cool my feet in the fresh river waters, while the sun warms my heart and soul. I feel the surge of her power flow through my body.

Tears threaten me all the while. Crying is something that I would be really embarrassed to do in front of strangers. Mad thoughts enter my brain. What if I started to cry and everyone joined in? I can visualise the scene in my head, all of us a mass convulsion of crying and a clatter of counsellors panicked, unable to control us all at once. I battle with reality and escapism but manage to clear my mind of madness and return on my journey of serenity and the calm of nature.

Our relaxation comes to an end and I come back to the room reluctantly, feeling refreshed and relaxed. I smile at the sleepy heads as they wake in wonder, oblivious to the hour that has passed. I realise that it was just what they need for today, space and an hour of sleep in the safety of others. I leave now, wishing for the week to pass so my mind can have its freedom again and I am grateful to have found this treasure, a place where I can clear the fog from my head.

I continue my classes through my illness on and off when I feel up to it, though they are regularly tainted with sadness at the passing of one of our friends. I stay, needing the security and understanding, but mostly the peace and calm in my mind.

We are also taught relaxation I use at night when I feel the world sleeps but for me. I find it a comfort; it helps me rest and deters negative thoughts that threaten to drag me to sadness and possibly a 'poor me' syndrome. I would hate myself if that happened.

**

Moments lost forever

Declan and I would usually be quite physical; not OTT, just the odd hug, more acts of fun than anything sexual but I sense now he is afraid; he worries he might hurt me in some way. So I watch like an outsider as our relationship becomes strained by concern and fear of the unknown. I can't blame his wariness: two scars on my neck, one on my chest; an alien instrument (Portacath) in my body; and, to top it all, cancer, along with a stern talking to by the doctor on the dangers of becoming pregnant. All this is enough to put even a nymphomaniac off sex for life. To be truthful, I too am afraid and mostly I lack the will. So that is that and, like the hours of our life, intimacy slips away unnoticed. It is strange that this is probably the first time in my life that I really need physical interaction and we just can't muddle through the mess and find the ease and effortlessness that existed between us before. I have no idea how long my treatment will last or when I will be well again. Minutes, seconds of lust and love are lost forever and ahead a struggle to be natural and normal with each other when the cancer has left our bed. Where will we begin?

***

6 May 2001

Back in hospital. I pray it will be a short stay. Today the ward is stifling. The sun burns through the huge windows. It doesn't help that one minute I feel roasting with aches and pains and the next a chill shoots through my system. My body starts to shake involuntarily and my teeth are chattering. It reminds me of happier days as a child in Finglas playing in the snow without the warmth of gloves. We were determined to bear the pain of frozen fingers and toes – snowfall was too good to miss and we knew too well it would only last a short spell. But here I am now, an adult, lying scared, teeth chattering uncontrollably. I become dizzy and my head pounds. I lie unmoving, drifting in and out as the faces of my family click before me like a slide show: Declan, click, my mother, click, my sisters, click. Declan sits beside me now. The ward is quiet. I have a sudden memory: one of the girls had been told there is no more hope for her and a blanket of grief covers the ward. And with a blink I am gone again.

I talk to Declan, telling him how I feel, but he tells me later that he never heard me utter a word. My mind plays games with my mouth. I feel very weak and a pain in my chest and back are cause for concern. An x-ray machine is brought to the ward, as I am too ill to sit. We seem to be prone to clots and I assume this is what they are looking for. I have no will for further thoughts.

I doze in and out of consciousness and, when awake, I feel unnerved and out of control. I contemplate death. I know if I were to die now it would be easy, peaceful, a quiet passing. I think it would not be so bad. I would know no difference. I would be gone quietly and for some reason all fear of death seems to disappear. I wake fitfully; my eyelids weigh of lead. In a squint I check that Declan is still there. The ward is a background of muffles. I hear one of the girls ask her visitors to move outside. I hear my name. Maybe this is the end. Where is Graham and my family? I would like them here. I fade again to a nowhere, to a strange abyss. Perspiration runs down my face. I look for water and a fan to cool me. I must be bad – I already have one and they are in short supply and usually passed in consideration to those most in need. My body shakes uncontrollably and I lie staring round the room. I shiver, chilled now to the bone. I need some attention. I am frightened. Declan calls the nurse and in what seems like seconds a doctor arrives. A drip is attached and antibiotics are pumped to my cells. I am unaware of night or day. I wake. My mother sits by my bed. I sleep.

Today I wake. I am weak but feeling a little better and from now, day by day, I grow stronger. It seems I have septicaemia or sepsis.* Once again I have been lucky. My Portacath is deemed to be the host for the infection. I am not surprised. I have had people touch it without changing gloves having aided other patients. I have had young doctors brought from Accident and Emergency in the small hours of the morning to attach or detach me from my treatment and I have watched as staff pushed commodes and then directly attended me. I am angry – I could have died a stupid, pointless death, not of cancer but an unnecessary illness that could have been avoided by simple hygiene procedures! I wonder how many patients have spent months being strong, being brave, putting every last morsel of faith and hope into a treatment that racks our bodies, sheds our hair, sucks every last ounce of energy from our bodies and then died from this pathetic, stupid illness. God, I am angry!

***

Some of the nurses are brilliant the way they keep up the fun and craic even though it must get to them sometimes. Some of the girls have great understanding, especially those who have had family members with cancer at some stage. Most of the time you are treated with great respect but unfortunately, like in every walk of life, some people have no compassion or regard for their fellow human beings and let their ego get in the way. I think it is easy to forget that patients are human and sometimes are shown little respect when they are always lying down looking up to you, in pyjamas, totally dependent, so fragile and frail.

This may sound funny but it is true. I'm used to wearing a suit every day to work and it makes me feel in control and confident. Without clothes we are vulnerable and needy and

---

* A serious illness caused by overwhelming infection of the blood stream by toxin-producing bacteria.

with no identity; add terrified to that and you are like a baby left in the woods, unprotected and frightened. If you are unlucky enough to come across a doctor or nurse with a big ego and no patience you are in trouble and if you are like me and believe it is your right to know what is happening to you and question your well-being they will hate you every time.

***

Today opening my eyes is a chore. I am thirty-nine but feel a hundred and thirty-nine. I have been feeling really sick for the past few days. I make a huge effort and ask to sit in a chair. I think I am pushing it but I need to move. I need to leave this bed. I hate the restriction. I feel like a prisoner stuck in a nightmare alien world. I want to be well. I want to be free.

The doctors come. I know my blood levels are very low, but other than that I find most of the bedside medical chatter is going over my head. Normally I would have a question, say something to feel a part of my treatment, but today I am weary and silent. I hand my life freely over to the professionals. Today I have no will.

I am back in bed. I am weak and fear sees his chance. He comes to visit and stays well into the night. I stare into the darkness, my mind filled with thoughts of doom. I feel my body stoop and I try to straighten but with no impact. On days like this I wonder will I see my world again, will I have another chance to be part of this wonderful life. Or is this my end?

It is decided I must have a blood transfusion and platelets. I know I have a rare blood group and worry that there won't be a match available.

A doctor has taken personal offence to my family asking if they could give their blood to me direct. It appeared the hospital were having trouble getting me blood and platelets, and in their desperation my family, unknown to me, had asked an apparently really stupid question and worst of all had used the wrong chain of command. Their vital mistake was asking a nurse, who in turn told the doctor of their enquiry. For some reason, never explained to me or my family, the doctor came flying into the ward telling me of her speciality and that she would be handling anything to do with my blood, not the nurse. My family wanted to confront her about the obvious misunderstanding and their concerns but I begged them not to. After all I would have to meet this bully in the ward the next day, not them. My family were left with feelings of total inadequacy and foolishness and in their innocence all they had intended to do was help save my life.

I am drained in more ways then one and to be honest I feel a little blue. I let worry enter my head and he stirs negative thoughts. I have seen others become weak and it has been the beginning of their journey's end. I feel my heart race. She is running breathless in terror. I try to calm her. I try to be strong. I want so much to be well, to once again spend wonderful times with my precious family, to share laughter and fun with my friends. I just want to live.

A very important 'thank you'

The next day and good news – they have found a match. I feel the joy of all the Christmas morning gifts combined in one. This gift more precious than my life's worth of gifts and its very sight stirs a will, a desire to be, to live, and I feel a new respect for my fellow humans, who care, who want to help.

I lie in the bed watching the blood flow entering my body and I think of its journey from one being to the next. I feel my eyes well with overwhelming gratitude for the soul who took the time to care, to carry out a wonderful, selfless act of giving, giving to save a life. I wonder whose blood flows with mine but I know for sure it is that of a kind and caring human. I watch my veins and imagine them filling, swelling with this gift of life. I think of my unnamed Saviour. I wonder who you are? I lie here wanting so much to thank you, so I whisper to the world a wish of love and well-being for your life and hope an angel will catch it and carry my wish and sprinkle a mist of joy and peace on your world, so you may enjoy a healthy, happy life. Giving blood is a simple deed but it is life for me.

***

Through the sadness we somehow still manage to have such a laugh sometimes, especially as our treatment tends to get in sync with each other. Sometimes the whole ward is filled with friends visiting, so there is bound to be some messing. We are all advised against eating takeout food, as we are very vulnerable to any bugs or infection. Also, alcohol is as a no-no, but hey! this is not Temple Street and we are all adults. Plus we all know that people are enjoying their weekends and life is still going on outside – romantic dinners, parties with friends, weddings, birthdays, all the social interaction others take for granted – and we miss it all. People pass outside on the street at night singing and roaring, reminding us life is still in full swing. So if we all feel well enough, as some form of compensation we will order a Chinese or Indian. We will get it delivered or force some unfortunate visitor to collect it for us, leaving them worrying that they might be responsible for killing us all. But how can you argue with six bald, determined women? Karen always has a bottle of wine hidden somewhere as a treat and, I believe, purely for devilment. How could you deny her? She is only twenty-one and missing out on so much of her life.

To be truthful, the food is never eaten with great gusto and the wine shared by six is barely in the glass. But a great pretence is always made. I know it is just the normality we all long for, not the food or wine. It is the break in the stifling routine we hate so much that makes our adventure so great.

How easily pleased we are! On one occasion one of the girls was too ill to partake but begged us to do it as a distraction from her illness, anything for some form of normality. What a change lying in bed with the background noise of stifled laughter and whispering of fun – the best medication some of us get all day. We seize the nights and days when we are well, as the gloom returns all too quickly. One lumbar puncture or bone marrow test is enough to quieten us all.

***

The lost patient

A nurse's aide is always on hand if we need any daily help. She is run off her feet, just like the nurses. A lot of her time is taken every day with Lucy, an elderly lady who lives on the ward. Someone told me she has been there nine months. She stares at us confused and terrified, and I pity her with only an elderly sister to visit. She spends her days going in and out of the toilet, each time locking herself in and then banging the door for us to try to get her out. She never speaks. She only seems to grunt and I wonder was this always the way. She takes our magazines and glares at us if we try to sneak them back. Usually we leave it be. What is the point in upsetting her? It is as though she exists in another world and I have to admit she frightens me. Some days she tries to strip off all her clothes. We call to her but she stares back, her eyes wild with terror. We dare not approach. I feel so sad for her yet I am disgusted by her, and then I feel guilty. Who was she? If she could see herself here, sitting in a chair at the top of the ward, nappy removed and emptied on the floor, playing its contents around on the ground with her toe. She roars if we dare go near her. We call for the nurses but, as usual, they are all busy. We press the panic button. I hate the way the responder always asks, 'What is the nature of your alert? What do you need a nurse for?' In an emergency we all roar together, 'Can you just get us a nurse?!' It angers us all having to explain why we have pushed the button. The nurse arrives and guides Lucy to her bed. She shuffles her away behind the curtain and everyone relaxes again.

I am repulsed and afraid of the unhygienic mess she makes. Most times she misses the toilet and destroys the floor and wall. Usually whoever goes in next cleans as best we can so we can at least use the loo. Unfortunately for us on chemo, most times our toilet needs give little warning. Other days we ask that the cleaners come back on duty and clean the mess. I find again my heart growing angry at a government that leaves its aged and senile dumped in wards where they are frightened and degraded. I see Lucy's elderly sister, her heart breaking as she sits silent beside her and I feel ashamed of myself for the fear and disgust I hold for a woman who knows no better. I watch her sister try to make contact, searching, I suppose, in Lucy's eyes for a glimmer of her sister, the lost person.

I feel Lucy should be cared for with patience and kindness, in a place where staff have the time and experience for her needs; not on a hospital ward where she goes ignored most days. Her only activity appears to be the movement from bed to chair and back. I watch as we grow to despise her, week after week, when she wakes us from our already restless sleep. I see her eyes glaring at us with hate in her confused mind and I watch as our eyes reflect her look. We are worried sick of infection. We clean the toilet and door handles with antiseptic wipes, protecting ourselves as best we can. We are always nervous, as the chemo depletes our immune system, leaving us open to all types of killer bugs, and we are all too aware that an infection could get us first, robbing our cancer of its chance to kill us.

My feelings towards Lucy cause me great concern. I feel scared of her, yet upset for her. I watch her one day sitting legs spread, gown askew, nappy missing again. Our visitors avert their heads, confused in embarrassment for her and themselves. My heart breaks for her and I find then in a sick twist of morals I am glad for her that she knows no different.

Karen

Karen is twenty-one and, it seems, full of life. She is headstrong and determined. We have lots of laughs. One day Karen and I are having our usual hospital corridor stroll. We spot a notice pinned on a board informing us there will be a relaxation session downstairs. We return to the ward excited with the news and with the intention of gathering a clatter of wearied patients to participate. Unfortunately when we ring the number it turns out they can only accommodate two, so Karen and I are elected as guinea pigs. We find the room, a nice quiet place off the beaten track. There are two beds set up and a shy young girl struggles to get some music going on a tape deck. It is awkward, and Karen and I raise our brows in mute confusion; what do we do – lie, stand or sit?

Eventually we lie down and the gentle music floats through the air. The girl speaks in whispers, telling us to close our eyes and breathe deep breaths, in and out, while soaking in the calm, gentle music. I find the peace and break in our mundane routine relaxing and I close my eyes and try desperately to unwind and clear my mind. It is hard in the hospital setting to relax. Maybe given a few sessions we could learn how to defy our surroundings and unwind some more. I ask Karen on the way back up in the lift what she thought and if she had relaxed. I can't believe her response! We roar laughing all the way up in the lift – curious onlookers must have assumed we had lost the plot. You see, Karen's treatment has caused damage to her ears so her hearing is not great, and with the music combined with the whispering voice she had spent the whole time with one eye open trying to watch my every move in case she missed something. It was to be her first relaxation class and her last. It caused her more frustration than peace and left her totally peed off. Needless to say there was no getting her to do a class again and, on return to the ward, she put everyone else off, the little wagon.

Karen was happy. She sometimes escaped from the hospital and met some friend to go to a picture. She always brought us back little cheering-up gifts. She smiled. She cried. She lost her temper. She fancied a guy. She snuck off to town for an hour or two. She lived. She seemed so healthy but inside her blood was infected. Her life ended too soon. She is no more.

I have thought of this quite a bit lately. 'You will never have your combined wealth of love shown more than on the day you are born and on the day you die.' It is the only time when all who will truly love you come together and their love unites. But why can't we love each other every day the way we would love when we hear someone has limited time left? We all know that our time in this life could end any second of any day! I know that sounds very morbid but this is where my thoughts have gone, the way my mind now roams. I have started to question humanity. I remember with sadness the final months of Karen's life.

When she was here in hospital she had the maximum of two visitors a week, if she was lucky. Most nights she sat with her headphones on while our visitors came, bearing gifts and chatting. We did our best to include her as she read and re-read the CD covers in embarrassed distraction. Sometimes she left the ward and wandered the corridors alone to pass visiting time. She spent so much time in hospital, months and months on end. I had heard her personal family life was complicated and her young friends I suppose were too busy having fun to give a half hour to think of visiting the sick or dying.

But what makes me really mad was what happened when she died and the events at her funeral. The whole town was at a stand still. Roads were blocked. Shops closed. Two rows of school girls formed a guard of honour for her to pass through. A police escort led her on her final path. The chapel burst with its holy, its doors too narrow to accommodate us as we crammed together, flocking to say our final goodbyes. The cold stone tiles were now a floral carpet of guilt and grief. I wanted so much to run to the pulpit and push the priest aside and roar to the world: 'Where were you when she needed you?' My heart pounded and Righteousness raced in my brain, goading me to do her work. 'Go on, you could plead insanity. They will see the bandanna and know you have cancer. Do it. Do it quick. Karen would want you to do it.' But I couldn't, the coward I was. Righteousness withdrew and then I felt compelled to run, to leave this church and this ritual I no longer wanted to be part of. I wanted so much to get away. I felt trapped in a charade of shame.

So I left with disgust heavy in my heart, feeling disappointed in humanity and the greed with which we guard our twenty-four hours. I was consumed with sadness at the little thought we really have for one another and how we hide deep the disinterest we truly feel. As crowded as the funeral was, the next day life goes on and days pass and only the loved ones sit day after day solitary and lost with memories now their only remnant. The body of this special person now gone forever, they must rely on the past, replaying memories over and over until they can bear no more.

***

Religion

Over the months religion has often been a topic of discussion between us on the ward. The visit of a priest to some and minister to others usually stirs these discussions. The bell rings in the morning when the Eucharist has arrived on the corridor and mass goes on every day somewhere in the building. Religion hovers always around the hospital; you can sense its presence. For me there is no running back to a church I attended once a year at Christmas with family, or for attendance at funerals, weddings or other services that sporadically took me to her door. I keep my God in my heart.

Today I decide to attend mass, wanting an escape from the ward more than anything else. So I take my drip stand and we travel downstairs. It is a strange collection, the walking wounded squashed together, some left to stand, some balanced against doors. I am reminded of a war camp. It seems as though bandages and ailments are displayed on every conceivable part of the human body. Patients with black hollows below their eyes, some wizened creatures barely alive it seems, all praying in unison. I feel moved and when the prayers are spoken for all our well-being and recovery I feel my throat tighten and my eyes fill. I won't venture there again. It makes me sad.

It is early morning and as usual stillness descends on the ward. It is a time when we all lie quiet for different reasons. Some rustle morning papers. Others, drained, having slept little, doze contented now as we watch for them. Others too ill to know the difference between night and day rest peacefully. We have heard on the news and read in the papers that the pilgrimage of St Therese of Lisieux has come to Ireland. And I have received a pile of prayers in her honour, prayers given with hope that I will have a miracle, that I will be cured. I am appreciative for the wish for well-being that they bring. I lie outside the covers reading a magazine, dozing on and off. I wake to silence and the vision of what could only be described as a nun from the seventeen hundreds standing before me in the ward. She is still and silent, and serenely she turns without comment and walks from the ward. I sit startled, blinking in disbelief, not sure if I have woken or remain asleep. I scan the ward in urgency to see who else is alert and I see Jane sitting in bed, her newspaper held straight, head tilted, mouth open and she smiles and says, 'Please tell me you saw what I saw.' We laugh with nerves but contented – we are united in our vision. I can only assume that a nun from the Therese of Lisieux community took time to pay a quiet visit to our sleepy ward.

***

16 May 2001

I'm home again after ten days in hospital. It's great to be here – I really thought this time I might not make it. I go for lunch in the Gresham with the women from the relaxation class. I had decided today to try an eyebrow pencil. I needed to draw a line of judgement for my eye shadow – otherwise where do you stop? Just after lunch I go to the ladies only to discover that I have at some stage during lunch wiped one eyebrow off. I look ridiculous but we have a good laugh! I realise this one eyebrow look will probably be something of a regular occurrence for me.

What do we look like to the observing eyes? A colourful display of tomboy hair growths, wigs, scarves and bandannas. And there we sit, a circle of hope, bravery and respect, sharing stories of life. Susan is there – Annette has kidnapped her from the hospice. I remember Susan's pride. She insists that she will buy the wine, South African, in memory of some time she spent living there. We chat casually, our conversation tainted by the painful awareness that it will probably be the last time we see her.

***

My faith (a short story)

I was thirty-nine with a death sentence looming and needing some serious divine intervention. I was reared in a Catholic home where we knelt together for rosary and where silence fell unquestioned at the first dong of the Angelus. God, my Mam must have loved the twenty seconds of peace when six children sat frozen in time. I also went to mass every Sunday and until I hit my teenage years never challenged this practice, even though I hated the repetitiveness and would gawk around the church watching for any distraction. Sometimes I would spot a girl from school: we could carry out a conversation through our eyes and my lip reading wasn't bad either. My favourite part of the mass was, 'Go in peace to love and serve the Lord.' I responded, 'Thanks be to God' with such relief and filed from my seat wishing I could just climb over the back or push the old lady in front who was moving too slow. I can hear your murmurs of disgust but that was how I felt. I continued with mass until I was a teenager, when I began to cause a lot of hassle in our home on Sunday mornings. Then one day my brother took me aside letting me in on a very clever plan: 'Why don't you pretend to go to mass and just get a missalette from someone on your way home?' You see, it would be imperative that we had this information as my father was known to break into open debate about the mass content. Apparently my brother had been doing this for years, a great solution to our problem. But here I am now with cancer and no easy solutions.

One afternoon my uncle phoned me asking if I would take a trip to see a man renowned for his healing. I was afraid, as I had never experienced anything like that before, but my fear of death was stronger. Early one morning we made our journey to Galway. Busloads of people poured into the country church, those in wheelchairs taking front-row position. I stared around nervously, wondering why exactly I had come. The healer arrived and people began chanting in unison prayers I had heard as a child but whose words were long forgotten. I waited for hints to sit, kneel or stand, like a game of Simple Simon. I felt people's eyes burn into my back as they spotted the fraud amongst them. I knew that God would also be watching. Would he see me as an intruder, showing up years later begging for a favour? It was time to queue before the altar. My uncle progressed ahead, shuffling on his stick, announcing as he moved, 'She has cancer'. I wished that I could just evaporate and disappear forever as people parted to let me through.

The healer passed before the crowd, touching them along the way; they then collapsed into waiting arms and lay dishevelled before the altar. Even nuns lay there, skirts in disarray above their knees. He was getting nearer and my chance to run had evaded me. My heart pounded so loud I wondered could others hear it. He was before me now, 'Where is your cancer?' I don't remember speaking just pointing, determined that no matter what happened I would not fall. He placed his hands upon me mumbling words, eyes closed, evoking his power to heal and I stood my ground. He whispered, 'I will see you again' and in my heart I said, 'Not if I can help it!'

We drove home in silence, weary from our day. Maybe my uncle hoped he would look in the mirror and see me seated behind him, fresh faced, glowing with health. I wished for that too. When home I thought about my life. I remembered that there was someone I had always turned to in times of want, it was so subtle I had forgotten. If I lost an item I left it to my friend to find; when in doubt I asked his advice. He was always there for me and my faith in him was undisputed. Without doubt I knew St Anthony would find a way.

***

I had a conversation with a lady recently who couldn't believe how I thought a ward of cancer patients is better than a mixed ward, but for me without the girls I would have curled into a cocoon and I would not have had the chance to air lots of questions and doubts, and would not have met the most wonderfully strong people who changed me forever. If there is any joy in our hospital stay it is in knowing one or more of these friends will be in the ward when you arrive. It makes our time here somewhat bearable.

On the rare occasion when I see tears – brought on by a poor scan result or a long painful day for one of us – we all seem united in the suffering and a curtain will be pulled and muffled weeping will be heard. It is easier in my experience to handle our emotions if it is only cancer patients on the ward. The difficulty is when someone is just in for a couple of days for something routine. Something happens those days on the ward; it is as though a pause button is pressed on our feelings. There is less conversation and a crack forms in the support we give and get from each other.

One day we witness a nurse reassuring a very distraught non-cancer patient that they definitely do not have cancer and it is purely because there is a bed shortage and no designated cancer ward that she is placed on this ward with us. I am often so annoyed at visitors to non-cancer patients who bring kids onto the wards and let them run riot. Or the family of an eighty-year-old heart patient who brought two cakes at different stages during the day and sang 'Happy Birthday' over and over. I was so ill that day and it was torture. I just wanted to sleep or just even rest. I don't blame these families. The children are entitled to see granny or mammy, but when it is just cancer patients on the wards there is an understanding, like a list of invisible rules exists in relation to noise, mobile phones. A genuine concern for each other prevails and an awareness of how tired, sick and strained someone can be from chemotherapy.

It is strange now for me to remember my first days on the ward. I recall crying and begging my family not to leave me. When I saw the bald heads, bandannas, wigs and very sick people I couldn't understand why I was there and wanted to be anywhere else in the world. My mind couldn't seem to register what was really happening to me. I suppose I was consumed with shock. So can you imagine what it is like for non-cancer patients to be on this ward? You would need to be very strong.

***

Planning ahead

I was at a friend's funeral on Saturday, one of the girls, a friend I made in hospital. Like most of the women's funerals I had attended, it was packed. People cried and cried. There didn't seem to be a dry eye in the house, me included. I was thinking about my own funeral and imagined there would be a large number of people there whom I would never have met, people who work with my five siblings, with my father, with my son, with my partner. Also people I had not seen in years, some I worked with maybe years ago, possibly some old school friends and neighbours, friends of my family and my boyfriend's family. Some would probably cry. But why? Some would have no connection to me personally or any feeling of real loss, so why cry? At the funeral on Saturday I feel most of the people were crying for Catherine's parents, her two young children, her brother and sisters now that she is gone. I think people also cried for the shortness of life lived. Catherine was a young mother and it just seemed so unfair that she should not have the chance to live her life in full. Because she was so brave and fun-loving and took her illness head on, over and over again, there was a huge sense of sadness at her battle's end. Undoubtedly, her family and close friends love her and miss her and need to express it. But I still find it strange, the gathering of strangers who cry in unison for someone they never knew. I suppose it stirs in them a memory of a past personal loss.

Now that I have faced death and spent hours thinking about it, I think of my funeral. I feel, yes, do cry, but I would want some joy, maybe some stories told by family and friends of my wonderful life that I had been blessed to have. If the situation had been that I was in pain and with an incurable illness, I would like my release to be celebrated and everyone to be strong knowing I would never be too far away. It would be sad that the body I was supplied with let me down and that there is no modern solution that allows for transplanting a soul or spirit and so I must move on and be somewhere else. I love life so much and the thought of losing it is terrifying. I feel sick even writing this, but I must believe there is something somewhere special. But nothing that I could conceive in my head would make me want to trade the life I have now, a wonderful son, boyfriend, family and the brilliant friends I have been lucky to have. Unless, of course, I was in pain, lying in hospital day after day, going through what I already know would be in store for me. I would not be living the life I know, but some nightmare, some horrible existence and surviving as a person that can no longer be me and, yes, I would want to be released, yes to death, yes to freedom and maybe the possibility of a new beginning. Is that not cause for some joy?

***

23 May 2001

I am due in for the next lot of five-day chemotherapy, but there is no bed. Here we go again, more days of unnecessary extra stress and worry. The notion that the wait will start again is too much to bear. I am feeling blue today. I wake and sadness slaps me in the face and in a sleepy haze, I can't remember why. Am I awake? Is this a nightmare I cannot shake? My hand flies to my head. I panic for my hair and struggle from the bed, stomach churning, disappointed at this day, wishing with all my heart I could change the events of my life.

***

25 May 2001

I am admitted today, but I have to wait until 28 May for my fifth session of chemotherapy. Thank God it was only two days' wait for a bed this time.

I had a bad night last night. I was feeling really weird and had a sick stomach. I felt as though I might pass out at any second or just faint as I lay in bed, like a drain of everything from my body. It is really strange and the feeling unnerves me.

It is a beautiful day outside today. The heat in the hospital stifles any happiness and it angers me. I am smothering in this place. I want so much to go home. I feel like a little kid; I want to cry to my family. 'Please help me. Take me home.' I can't bear to be here. Instead I wander the corridors escaping the ward. Everyone on the ward seems very ill today. No one can muster a smile. I find myself in Outpatients and I watch the queues with envy. I listen to their words of anger; anger at the long wait, the hours of boredom, moaning out loud, 'This is a bloody disgrace! I am here since nine this morning.' 'Jesus, you're lucky. I had to travel from Dundalk and I am up since five.' I want to scream: 'Oh shut up! At least you will be in your house tonight lying with your loved ones, safe in your head and home. Take our places today, come up the stairs, see how others will spend their day.'

I want normality for even one hour. I long for the end of this nightmare. But at least here walking the corridors I feel human, I feel part of the world. I stroll back through the clinics and find an exit to the convent. There is a nip in the air when I wander from the sunshine and I shiver. I am not one for being conventional. I like to challenge, to break the rules, so I take a chance and continue on, curiosity holding my hand

and walking with me. We wander towards the convent grounds. What is the worst-case scenario? A nun will tell me I am trespassing and ask me to leave? I don't care. I shuffle on and then I find it – a secret garden! I sit on a sun-drenched bench, soaking its heat to my body and heart, and I listen to the birds as they carry on about their day. My ears broaden their horizon and I hear the manic traffic beyond the wall, where life continues without me. I wander slowly around, soaking in the beauty of each flower, each tree, each a wonder in the world I now belong to. I sit still for a long while, at peace for the first time in ages. Selfishly, I decide this will be my secret, my place for calm and joy. I return to the ward a happier person. I am so glad to be still alive. Once more I resolve to myself that I will live. I have to. I love this world and my life.

***

My Granda lived in Australia when he was diagnosed with cancer and my mother went out to visit him. On her return she told us of these beautiful communal kitchens where patients can help themselves when they felt up to it and in the humour. It must be wonderful to have the choice and not expect your stomach to eat breakfast just after you spent a night throwing up or spend all morning waiting for scans and drinking litres of white chalky solution only to be greeted on your return with a plate of fish, white sauce and vegetables. It should be up to you when to eat – most of us on the ward never ate the food anyway. Imagine also having the normality of supper and chats when you can't sleep. Now that is some form of homely pleasure we would have loved and, for long-term patients, a much more pleasant way to have to cope with months of treatment. In Australia they also had a garden and conservatory for long-term patients to relax and have a break from their bed. But who am I kidding – on occasions we don't even have beds for patients to start treatment, so how far down the list would the consideration be for the patients' struggle for sanity and calm?

June 2001

I feel really sad today, yet the ward is full of fun and joviality. There is a big Gaelic match on the TV and between visitors and patients we have a good mix of harmless rivalry. The sun is beaming its bright rays of heat into our ward and I find its presence is misplaced. I am sad, I am angry and I cannot shake this dark mood. Rita, another patient, a friend to me now, has received very bad news. The usual, the dreaded words: 'Sorry there is nothing more we can do for you.' She is a young mother with a daughter of three years. I see the sadness in her eyes but I see her face of bravery as her family visit. I want to scream to God, 'Why? Why this wonderful girl full of fun and spirit?' And I know I would hear no response from the skies or clouds, no voice would give me an explanation. I think of her mind and how it must struggle to comprehend these words of doom. I feel I cannot talk to her today. I fear I will bawl into her face and I would hate myself for that weakness in her circle of strength. I turn from her now as her baby runs to her and her husband kisses her lips. I hastily leave the ward and walk the corridor as tears fall from my eyes. I feel so ashamed, guilty and angry. What right have I? What the hell am I crying for? I feel I could punch myself for being so pathetic. I live, my news still arrives positive in staggered snippets. Why should I cry? I cry for her because I know how I would feel: my heart would break in one quick snap like a stick beneath my feet if

I thought I must leave my child, my family, my life. And once more I am reminded today that death has brushed her lips against my face, but she has spared me her kiss.

Visiting time is over and the ward breathes still and peaceful. Rita calls me to her bed. My heart beats in panic and I whisper to my eyes, 'Please don't cry, please don't cry', over and over like a mantra as I baby-step my way to her. She asks me how my scan results were. I want to lie to her, to tell her I will also die and then we could unite in grief, unite in understanding, but instead I tell her the truth with a shaky voice, 'All is fine.' She smiles a genuine face of delight. I talk crap for a few minutes as my tongues wags with nerves. I feel her sense this and I stop. I ask how she feels and she talks with no nonsense in strong understanding of someone who has accepted their lot. We talk about life and death, and I listen to her medical record as though she were a consultant. She talks of how she will spend her final days and her hopes for her daughter's future and with bravery and acceptance she says, 'You know they told me from the start I never really had much hope; it was always just a little hope.' And I want to scream. I wish with every speck of my being that I had one wish, one miracle – I know I would use it this minute. And then she looks sad and says the strangest thing: 'Janette, you know the way you believe you can be well if you completely set your mind to it?' I nod. 'And your faith in St Anthony?' I nod again. 'Well,' she asks me with a grin, 'Can you do what you do for yourself for me?' I look to her, my sorrow and sympathy no longer hidden, and I reply, 'Rita, if only I could, if only.'

**

Doubt is testing me today. She sneers at my beliefs and my dreams and questions my philosophy. I feel the weakness but I know it is my fear for Rita that allows doubt the freedom to scan my brain and scatter her seeds of uncertainty into my thoughts. And she succeeds, her words determined and precise: 'What if you are wrong? Maybe you too will die like the others. Maybe you are fooling yourself through fear. Maybe St Anthony never even lived and mind over matter is a load of tripe. What if positive thinking is only a way to stop you from losing your mind?' And the rant goes on and on until I feel myself slip and I pull my curtain and let the silent tears flow. I stay quiet for a while, just sitting still. A floral curtain of cotton separates me from a room of lives and none of us knows our future. I slowly calm with acceptance and eventually I pull myself together. I gather my beliefs once more and I encase them in a wall of strength, hiding them in a place I know they will be safe and I leave them secure in the knowledge that Logic is guarding them.

I walk along the corridor. I need some space. It is a bad week: another one of the girls has been told her treatment has not worked and that there is no more they can do. As I walk by her ward a friend of hers speaks to me. I enquire about her pal, 'How is Joan today?' And she replies with heavy words of gloom, 'She is dying, you know?' And for some reason I reply, 'I know, but how is she?' It struck me I had learned a wonderful lesson from Rita that until that last breath, we are who we are – life is lived in nanoseconds and each one matters to you, especially when you are counting.

***

1 June 2001

I am allowed home today. I will be glad to get home to my little house. It has been a long, hot seven days on the ward. Mam and Dad are coming to collect me. Dad will wait in the car as parking is a nightmare. He usually tries to get a space as near as possible in the temporary parking spaces as most times I am very weak and would not be able for a long walk.

It can take a few days before I build some strength up again. I sit waiting on the bed, dressed since early morning ready to escape. We never seem to break this ritual. If we are told at eight in the morning we can go, we all rush to dress and pack our bag, though we know it could be hours before we get our discharge letter and prescription and eventually exit the building. I think we fear something might happen to us and cause our leaving to be cancelled and if we're dressed we feel nearer the door. We just want out of here as soon as possible.

Mam walks onto the ward, happy to take me home. I stand to greet her and as I do a flush rushes down my leg, pours along, soaking my trousers and on to the floor. The fluid runs, no warning, no sign – without even, it seems, the opening of my bowel. I stand rigid, tears of shame rush to my eyes. Someone calls a nurse and I am ushered to the bathroom. She tells me not to worry, they will clean things up, and asks how I am feeling. I tell her I have no pain and had no gurgling or warning of what was to come. Jane gives me a loan of new pants she has and I am lucky I have a spare tracksuit bottoms with me. I fret that this hiccup may mean I will no longer go home and I cry internally at the thought. But nurse wanders off and no mention is made of me staying. I get out while the going is good and head for home.

***

Theresa

I bring Theresa, one of my friends from the classes, to visit Susan, a mutual friend of ours, who is now in the hospice. Susan has been informed her life is now over and it is a matter of days, hours, minutes, who could tell? I feel for Susan, but I feel more for Theresa in a strange way. Theresa has lost her leg and is finding the world a struggle to get around. We chat on our journey of our fears and worries and our hope of life. But Theresa's chances are slipping away and her news is bad. I worry for her as we visit Susan, mindful that this could be her next move. Were we hospice hunting, like visiting a show house on a lazy Sunday afternoon? Were we really checking out our options?

As we drive up to the hospice, I am anxious about what would greet us. To our surprise, it is not so bad – well, not so bad if you have no other choice. We find Susan resigned and waiting and my heart hurts. God, how can she cope when her options are now non-existent? The hospice is bright and airy, with a sense of life as opposed to death. There is freedom for patients to enjoy good days and yet have safety and care for the bad ones. Susan speaks to me of her fear to acknowledge her fate and my heart breaks for her. She has apparently always been a no-nonsense type of person but now she must face the challenge of her lifetime and sadly it is death. Another two wonderful ladies lost to their family and to this world.

***

My greatest fear now is fear of fear itself. I don't want to live in its shadow, to have fear always walking one step behind me waiting to be summoned. Is it waiting like a hunting cat ready to pounce at the first sign of weakness or distraction? I want to be free, to be myself, to stop thinking these deep thoughts of life and death. I want things to be as they were – work, home, weekends with family and friends – to live life full and happy. I don't want to think, will I see my grandchildren, will I have holidays or new experiences with family and friends? How long will I have? It's very hard not to think of these things when your brain has now explored new territory. It is so scary: one day your thoughts are on family, work, dinners, bills and the next your whole existence is in question. I just want to have casual thoughts of no importance, relaxed thoughts of silly, irrelevant, mundane, everyday things. I want my mind to be calm, to be at peace, but mostly, I want to be free.

***

6 June 2001: Neutropenic

I go to the clinic even though I know there are no beds. I am too ill to be at home: I need medical help. I attend the Day Clinic on the 6, 7 and 8 June. Three days pass and each day I gradually feel worse and worse. A combination of exhaustion, diarrhoea and low bloods leaves me wrecked and scared. I struggle from the car again. This time I am too ill to leave the hospital so they have no choice but to find a bed. I imagine they are forced to play God as they juggle us patients around hoping for the best. I feel guilty again, wondering who has missed their slot in this degenerated health system where a lottery is played with our lives or who has been evicted too early from their sick bed. I promise myself I will not let the guilt bring me down.

***

Sometimes we pass the time looking out the hospital window into the Mountjoy prison yard. It is a distraction watching the prisoners, us in our prison, them in theirs. Us locked up for months and pumped with a pharmacy of drugs and for no crimes. Some of the prisoners I am sure are pumped for their pleasure with a drug of their choice; our drugs are pumped to salvage a life. Us lying on death row, waiting, always watching as seasons pass. Parole for good behaviour is never an option for us. I grow jealous of them: at least they have some freedom and energy. We watch them in the yard playing ball, others walking in the fresh summer air as the sun warms their bodies, and here we stay, with no escape, weak, smothered, overcrowded, people everywhere and not a space for us to think. We have no reprieve from the sadness that consumes every vessel. Some days it is so strong I swear it has a scent.

I can't seem to clear my mind for one minute in this ward. There is one room we can go to. It contains a TV and video but they usually stand mute as the room mainly seems to be occupied by families doing bedside vigils; those not wanting to leave for fear they will miss that all-important final breath. These visitors will sit obscured in a fog of smoke, nerves, it seems, sending them into a chain-smoking frenzy. Their conversation is not something we want to hear. Plans of funerals and someone's passing and in their grief we sit invisible among them.

***

Ashling

Ashling, one the girls on the ward, was in serious trouble. (Well, how much more serious can trouble get than having a rare, incurable cancer?!) Apparently she did a runner from the hospital. She told me that herself and another girl snuck out to some pub in Dorset Street. There was murder. God, she had great spirit and basically didn't care what anyone thought. I got talking to Ashling a few times before she got too ill to speak and I now believe she was running from her future. She was very angry and at first she used to frighten me. But, like us all, she couldn't bear to face what was happening to her. She was full of rage and it was as though it oozed from every pore. One thing I don't understand was why she suffered so much pain. Every day open sores of raw skin were peeled from her body and repeatedly dressed and undressed. She screamed in agony. No one deserves that! I felt such pity for her.

Ashling had every reason to be angry. She was pregnant when she was diagnosed and during her treatment was taken to the Rotunda to have her beautiful baby. She returned the next day minus her son. To me it was like a ray of hope when her baby was brought over to see his mam. The whole ward was cheered by him. I let my mind dream as I looked in his perfect sweet baby face, us all cooing like idiots, each of us believing he signalled us out for a smile. I watched the baby's gummy grin of pure peace, the soft smell of innocence radiating from his velvet skin. A baby – to me the ultimate symbol of life – and he screamed his life to our ward.

I wondered could Ashling beat the odds and live for this little bundle of love. Maybe in another world, another life, but sadly not this one. I know Ashling had her problems before she was ill but her will to live was as great as anyone's.

***

16 June 2001

Eight days in my prison this time. God I miss my old life. Most days in the shower I still forget I am bald and I lift the shampoo and automatically pour it on my hand ready for use. It is a strange action, something I have done every other day for years and years. A motion without any prior contemplation and an act I have found so hard to break. Every time, this simple act brings with it a gripping sadness and an overwhelming reminder of how my life has changed. I wonder can you ever get used to having no hair. Besides the obvious coldness, you just don't look yourself. In the house with my family I remove the bandanna, but the ring of the door bell always causes a panic and I fumble for my bandanna to cover up.

***

Our first big night out in months. We go to our local for a quiet drink. I feel vulnerable; the noise is deafening, the crowd's laughter makes my insides flinch and I hate it all – the smoke, the chatter, the pushing sway of bodies as I venture terrified to the loo. Why had I come? I cannot believe I am so afraid, afraid of people, afraid of life.

***

I go again to a meditation/relaxation class. I need space and time out. I drift, feeling warm and safe yet surrounded by a group of strangers. Our facilitator speaks gently, relaxing us to a state of calm and peace. We are asked to picture in our mind a large box in the corner of the room and imagine that we place our troubles in it. She then continues with the relaxation technique that I really enjoy. We are eventually brought back to the room and, when ready, we are asked to take from the box what we had left there earlier. I am horrified by this, as I had left my cancer in the box and had no intention of taking it home. I wonder how many people do the same and never really understand why it is expected we take these woes with us when departing. I suppose in truth every time I go I leave more and more of my cancer behind without any realisation that I am doing it. If only it could be done in one go, wouldn't that be wonderful?

***

25 June 2001

I am due back in hospital today for my sixth session of chemotherapy – a five-day course. I wake strong and resolved. If there is no bed I will not crumble. I will not sit whimpering this time; I will do something, I will fight. I phone the hospital – 'Sorry, no bed' – and so the nightmare begins again. This is the most appalling torture to any human. I wonder am I really alive or am I in a coma. I must have crashed or had some major accident. This is not really my life. It can't be. I will wake soon and all will be okay. I rub my arms – I need to feel flesh to know I am alive, to know I do exist. Maybe I have just died and gone to hell. 'Ours is not to reason why, ours is just to do or die' – I could never live by this code!

I have made a strong decision today and I will stick with it. I have decided I will not be treated like this. I will do what I can to highlight the issue of bed shortage. I must keep myself active, sane. I need to keep focused, to be strong, to know I will be okay. I email and phone all the radio stations outlining my story. The day passes without response. In desperation I ring my friend Aine Ni Bhrion who bought me the diary to record all my positive thoughts. How things have changed from listing positive thoughts to listing days of torment. She works in radio and has lots of contacts. I need her help. I need the story to be told. I know I am trying to find a channel for my frustration and anger. It must be used in a positive way. I need to keep my head together. Feeling sorry for myself is never an option.

***

Today I get a call from Joe Duffy from RTE radio. He is an old friend of Aine's and has heard of my previous delays in getting a hospital bed. He asks me to tell my story on the radio. In unison, fear and delight rush through my body. But this is what I wanted. There is no turning away. No change of heart. I am very nervous and I wonder what in God's name I am doing. What have I brought now to my family's door? But I think of all those too ill or nervous to tell of this extra suffering patients must endure. I find strength from God only knows where and I say yes, I will do it, I will break the silence and talk.

It is arranged that my other friend Ann Whelan will be on the other line, ready, waiting to take over if my voice fails. I start by telling the listeners of my illness and the horror of our nationwide hospital bed shortage. I am shaking and my voice quivers with stress. I feel my face and neck burn with anguish and anger. And I know it can't be good for me. But sitting stressed and useless at home waiting on a bed is worse. Every day I sit with no treatment I feel I sit waiting for death. And I want all the people in this country to know how cancer patients are suffering this extra torment. I tell of my frustrating daily calls to Bed Management and the wait for them to call me back if a bed is free. I try to be calm and strong, but when I tell of how it is affecting me I stop. My nerve has gone and I tell Joe I have to take a break. The tears flow and I must catch my breath. The weeks have caught up. I am angry at myself for crying. I want to do my best for everyone.

Thank God Ann Whelan is on the other line and steps in strong and clear to answer Joe's questions. She is wonderful and never misses a beat. I am grateful to her for her caring nature and her desire to help. I breathe deeply and control my emotions. I have one chance and I want to make the most of it. Joe comes back and asks if I am okay to talk again. I gather myself together and I tell him I am fine. I find I am embarrassed that I have cried on air. But my need to be heard is greater than my concern for self-image.

Next on the line is my sister Miriam and she speaks of our parent's concerns for me and also the upset and worry for the rest of our family. Again I breathe deep to control my tears. And then the radio station's phone lines go mad and the support beams through the airwaves. I am forever grateful to Tom, Betty, Brendan, Margaret, Josephine, Tracey, Mary, Gerard and others whose names I failed to catch. They give me strength as they tell their sad stories, all carbon copies of mine. I feel proud of us all, strong and united with a will to be heard, and we bond in pain and frustration

One man tells of his inventive idea. He feigns illness and goes in through A&E to get a bed so he can get back in the system and, most importantly of all, get his next lot of vital chemo. I smile in admiration and know that no one in the world would think he committed a wrong doing. A soft-spoken lady rings in and relays the guilt she feels, guilt at something beyond her control. It happened that she overstayed her time in hospital following an operation. She tells how she got an infection and had stayed in the hospital a week longer than what was first thought. I feel for her and interrupt her and we unite in guilt: my guilt that by creating a fuss I will skip the queue; hers that she feels she overstayed and stopped a cancer patient getting crucial treatment. I feel disgusted that this obviously sensitive, caring person should ever have to feel a worry for becoming ill and needing a hospital bed. And I feel disgust at a system that turns cancer patients into liars and creates hate, anger and guilt in our hearts.

Casually during the interview I mention our human right to life, our right to treatment and how I feel there must be some solicitor somewhere willing to take a case for our rights. I speak the words without real consideration. But later these words would spring to mind in a moment of desperation with nowhere else to go.

***

26 June 2001

I am still sitting and waiting for a bed but I am not alone: fear as always keeps me company. I have hours to ponder, hours that should be spent in fun and laughter. These could be my final days, my final hours. No one knows and yet I sit worrying – not about my cancer, no; I am forced to worry about getting my treatment. Treatment that I am told is needed urgently and in a planned schedule; treatment that was initially given urgent and essential as I lay in Intensive Care fighting for life. I think of all the hundreds of families affected each year by cancer and all those who have battled for a bed. I see my treatment and proper health service as a simple basic human right and I wonder what sort of a nation stays silent while their government ignores their sick and weak. I know in my heart my cancer is in the hands of God and I must wait. My job is to be strong and positive. I worry a day will come when I am too ill to fight, to speak, to care. I am weak now but my spirit is strong and my will to live oozes from every pore. I know while I have a voice and a functioning brain I can certainly do something to highlight this repulsive treatment of patients and their families. I resolve that I will not put up with this; I will find a way.

***

Taking action

Today I wake and Anger is with me again. We start our day not with breakfast but with a phone book, paper and pen. I make a list of people I could call, starting with Patients' Services. But they are no help. The ward: no help. Social Services within the hospital: a sympathetic ear and source of what I feel are pathetic stupid words: 'Try not to worry.' I gradually move down my list of numbers and I make call after call in frustration and despair. The Irish Cancer Society is unaware there is any bed shortage. I know they do great work in palliative care, but what are they doing for those of us who still have a chance at life? Yes! We could possibly need them in a month or so, but maybe not if they would help us now to get our treatment. For the following hours I hear a mantra, over and over, 'No bed, no bed, no bed'.

I try my best to think logically, but thoughts of death are more real now than ever. What damage is being done as I am denied my treatment, denied my saviour? I visualise the tumour slowly stretching out, curling from its mass, happy as its killer abates. I imagine it alert, gaining strength to take control again, to regain its ground. But as long as I can breathe and have strength it will not happen. However, I must face the reality: I am slowly running out of options, but I cannot bear to let my mind think that thought for long. If I have no options I think I will truly die. And then it comes to me as I sit dazed, flicking through the phone book, scanning its dead pages for help. Simple: *'My right to life'* – that's it! I have a right to life. I have a right to treatment. I feel everyone must have. But I need someone to help me, to guide me in my battle for 'my right'. I try a couple of solicitors from the phone book but with no result. I spend hours racking my brain for a channel, a way to find the help I need. Who will be brave enough to challenge the Department of Health, the State, the hospital? They would have to be strong and willing.

Eventually I phone a friend of mine who works in close contact with different solicitors and I ask for his help. True to form he gives me the number of a man renowned for taking chances and caring about real people with controversial cases. An appointment is made and after one meeting I know he is the one. A person who seems to care genuinely. I am frightened about the financial end of things: 'How much will this battle cost?' I have heard stories of people taking on governments and large corporates only to lose everything, including their homes. However, I am assured I will be kept informed and when any expense might be incurred I will be notified immediately beforehand. I feel vulnerable yet I feel I can trust him and let events just take their course.

Over the next few hours I am asked to write dates, times, every last piece of information since I first fell ill. And the strangest thing of all is I have held on to everything, even the receipts for payment for my first private consultant's fee. It is as though I looked into the future and knew that I would have cancer, be denied my treatment and need all this paper work. How odd.

Everything is moving so quickly. The next day my appeal is in the High Court. I am not required to attend and I am glad of that. I sit at home waiting for a call from my solicitor. I watch the clock and contemplate how life can change so fast, in the blink of an eye. All we know as safe and normal can be swept from under us in a split second and there is not one damn thing we can do about it. I find it hard to believe that somewhere in the city courts strangers speak of my life, my rights and my personal medical records. What do I want from this? I want to shame the government, the hospital, the State; I want everyone to know; I want change; but mostly I want to save other cancer patients going through the torture and misery I have suffered. My whole body is shaking from the inside out. My Mam sits with me. And then it happens, something I never expected, something I never even considered.

***

The media

They come foraging for a story. Phones ring over and over, mobile, landline. How do they know my number? Who knows? Then they come knocking, looking for the photos to humanise the story of the minute. I am terrified but I have started this and I will see it through. I watch the news in shock as my face flashes before me and I joke again about my timing to be on TV, definitely not looking my best. My injunction has been taken against the Mater Hospital, the Eastern Regional Health Authority, the Minister for Health and Children, the Minister for Finance and the Attorney General. I read the words in the paper 'CANCER MUM BEGS FOR LIFE' and feel very embarrassed. It is surreal. I cannot believe I have started this, but I will continue. They say one clap starts an applause and if this will help someone else then it will have been worth the added stress I have taken on. I wonder how long this problem of bed shortage has been going on, but mainly I wonder why we, as humans, let it happen. Most of the legal jargon goes over my head, but the bottom line in English is: 'Give her a bed and the chemotherapy she needs to live.'

***

Today one of the young doctors is really annoyed with me for asking questions. I think I am jumping too far ahead for his liking. He wants my brain to take the pace he desires. My questions for whatever reason must fester in his mind all morning because after a few hours he stomps onto the ward, my charts clenched in his hand, asks my visitors to leave, roughly swings my curtains back and bombards my head with paragraphs of information. He storms off in a temper, certainly leaving nothing to my imagination and even forecasting things that might never happen.

When he leaves me I cannot stop shaking. I steady myself enough to follow my visitors down the corridor, ignoring the girls in the ward as they call after me, 'Janette, are you okay?' Words of bone marrow transplant are spinning in my head as I ignore their question. They have obviously heard everything through the thin curtains. I stumble down the corridor needing to locate my waiting friends. I collapse into my pals and sob. And then in the confusion a voice says, 'Excuse me, are you Janette Byrne?' I turn to her with my eyes red and swollen, chest still consuming short gasps of air in an effort to regain composure and control. In a daze I reply, 'Yes, I am Janette.' A formal, officious voice responds, 'Hello Janette, I am from administration. I need you to fill out a Freedom of Information form. You have given your solicitor permission to access your files.' In my despair her words make no sense and I wonder is she mad. Can she not see my despair, tears running uncontrolled down my face, lungs struggling to control my breaths of sadness? Can she not see my friends as they try to comfort me, confused as they stand still, unaware what words of horror have been spoken to me? I see the terror in their eyes and I assume they fear I have heard the worst. I must ease their worry, but when I speak it is in sobs, incoherent words of no sense. I slowly calm myself and explain the barrage of unnecessary information unleashed on my ears.

***

Legal stuff

The High Court
Even the mention of my name on the reams of legal documents is enough to scare me.

> Notice of motion Janette Byrne on 27 June
> Between
> Janette Byrne
> and
> The Mater Hospital, the Eastern Regional Health
> Authority, the Minister for Health and Children,
> the Minister for Finance, Ireland and the
> Attorney General.

A snippet of information taken from reams and reams of legal documentation:

> An interim and/or interlocutory order of mandamus by way of an application for judicial review directing the respondents, the servants or agents to immediately make available to the applicant and her medical team the necessary medical resources for the treatment of Non-Hodgkin's Lymphoma.

It was submitted that there was a statutory imperative on the board to provide Ms Byrne with the necessary services for her treatment.

It was also submitted that Ms Byrne was entitled to her treatment because of her constitutional right to life and bodily integrity.

The ERHA representative stated, 'While her treatment was not something we could provide we are willing to write the cheque.'

***

Media coverage

Words scream from the pages and I sit with a coffee and read them as though they relate to someone else.

'PLEASE JUDGE SAVE MY LIFE'
'CANCER CASE SHOWS DAIL'S MORAL BARBARISM'
'NO BED FOR TERRIFIED CANCER MUM'
'DECISION TO CALL OFF CANCER TREATMENT UNACCEPTABLE'
'THE FIGHT FOR LIFE'
'THE NIGHTMARE OF CANCER, THE DARK REALITY OF THE HEALTHCARE SERVICE'

I cannot comprehend that they speak of me. I am mortified. I think of all my customers, friends of old, anyone who knows me or my family and I cringe with embarrassment. The reporters knock on my door again. I am drained; I can do no more today. I hear my mother telling them I am too unwell and too upset to talk today. I hear her polite chatter, protecting her child, and I think of the stress I have brought on all my family. I am sure some would say I am mad. Why bring this extra hassle on everyone? Given the chance, I would respond, 'Because all I have is my fight, my will to live and no one will stand in my way.'

I fluctuate between indifference and terror. My emotions are still a mess. I watch the news and my face stares back and I worry again about what I have done. Maybe the sceptics are right: maybe I am wasting my time and maybe no one cares. Soon I will know.

***

27 June 2001: High Court decision

It is decided that a place should be provided for me at the Mater Private if one is not available for me in the public hospital by Monday and the ERHA will pick up the bill. Justice Kelly states: 'One would have to have a heart of stone not to be sympathetic with Ms Byrne; she had eight hours in the operating theatre and an unfortunate history of post-op treatment.' And again the media bombard our world:

> 'VICTORY IN STRUGGLE AGAINST CANCER, JANETTE WINS COURT BATTLE FOR HOSPITAL TREATMENT'
> 'CANCER WOMAN WINS RIGHT TO TREATMENT'
> 'WOMAN WINS BATTLE TO GET CANCER TREATMENT'
> 'CANCER VICTIM TAKES FIGHT FOR TREATMENT TO COURTS'
> 'BLAME GAME IS REAL CANCER IN THE HEALTH SERVICE'

As I read the newspaper my first reaction is one of guilt. Who would be evicted to accommodate me? I also feel bad for the other girls at home waiting to get back into hospital, some waiting longer than me, some without family support and too sick to fight their own case. I want to take it all on; I want to fight their fight. I feel agitated that I don't have the strength but I know genuinely in my heart I cannot carry that extra burden at the moment. In truth I feel I have already taken on more than I can handle. If I go to the Mater Private on Monday I will be without my hospital friends, my support, my inspiration, and it will be a very long stay without them.

***

28 June 2001: Result!

As it happens a bed is made available in the Mater public. Surprise! Surprise! I arrive at the hospital on Monday. I have no idea what to expect. I have worried a lot about the staff and their reaction to me. What if they are angry? What if they ignore me? But I have forgotten something very important; the majority of the staff want to help us – they want to treat us, heal us. The bed shortage puts a strain on the never-ending conveyor belt of illness and, most importantly, they and their families are patients too and, if unfortunate, they will also have to use the system and I assume they don't get preferential treatment.

I walk sheepishly along the corridor waiting for a reaction, waiting for someone to ignore me or scowl in response to the sight of me. I see Joe and his daughter walking towards me. His wife Isobel has been moved to a private room. Her life is now counted in hours, minutes and seconds. I see his face creased with anguish and pain and I want to run. The corridor seems to lengthen and stretch for miles. He walks straight for me, hand extended, and in a shaky, choked voice says, 'Well done. Fair play to you.' He tells me that Isobel has had to endure nights on a trolley or sitting in a chair in the A&E and has also sat at home phoning day in and day out for her bed during her days of hope. He says that he admires me for taking a stand. I am touched by his words and my heart fills with gratitude. With that one handshake I feel relief flood through me. I need nothing else; for me now it has all been worthwhile and I no longer care what anyone else thinks.

I wander on to the ward, leaving Joe to spend his final moments with Isobel. I am greeted by an air of excitement as girls pass on words of encouragement and we talk for ages about our different horror experiences and how it affects us all. The nurses come at different stages through the day and while some do not comment, others air their support and admiration at my stance. I am elated and proud.

***

Today I am doing a radio interview from the hospital. I am not feeling the best: nerves, stress and chemo – not a good mix. Apparently the Minister for Health will be on the air and will be grilled about the bed shortage. I have never met or spoken to a Minister and I am very anxious. The girls on the ward are excited and keep asking me to say different things to him, to enlighten him of our plight. I find I cannot concentrate and at stages my mind goes completely blank. But at least today I know it is nerves and stress that cause the confusion in my thoughts.

The girls all gather in the day ward. A radio sits on the sill. The sun burns through the window and the ward is stifling. It is strange to see them all sitting in the recliner chairs, free, unattached and happy. It is here we come when we are brought from home with a problem or worry, here where day patients come and get their much-needed treatment. It is a room where quiet is the norm, where people sit pensive, reading or dozing as the drugs flow through their veins; a room where happiness seldom ventures. But today it is like a classroom of boisterous teenagers, giddy with anticipation at term's end. I watch their smiling faces of support and I know they relish the distraction. I want so much to do them proud. I want to make a difference. Who knows, I may not be here next month. What have I to lose besides my life? I will do this for the cancer patients to come. At least if we are all gone they will hopefully benefit.

I move away to a quiet room. My heart races in my chest. My face burns with a mix of anger, fear and panic. I want to abort the plan but it is too late. I hold the phone to my ear waiting for the programme to start. U2's song plays in the background, 'Stuck in a Moment' – how apt.

My pal Ann Whelan is in the Today FM studios and Fintan O'Toole, the presenter of the Last Word that day, begins by talking to her. I listen as she tells him my story from the beginning and how I was taken to hospital choking, my diagnosis of lymphoma and the added stress I and other cancer patients must endure trying to get a bed. Ann talks of the anxiety this has caused me and my family and friends. She speaks very clear and precise but I can hear her anger as she talks about our country that is awash with money, a country where a Celtic tiger runs fast and furious. I hear her disbelief that cancer patients are put through this torture at a time when we should be cared for with urgency and compassion. I am again grateful to Ann for her friendship. She was always the most outgoing of the group, the cheeky one, and I am glad today for her bravery and outgoing personality. Fintan says he wants to bring me in; my heart misses a beat, beads of sweat gather on my forehead and my breath is restricted with fear.

He thanks me for doing the interview from the hospital and asks me what it feels like to know you need treatment but not be able to get it. I tell him about the horrible ritual of phoning day in day out to see if a bed has been freed up, about how that upsets me so much. I explain how I had originally directed my anger at the girls in Bed Management and at the nurses and how wrong I had been. I was ignorant to the fact that bed shortage is a country-wide problem and that these people have no control, no options. I speak of how angry it makes me that cancer patients are treated in this way and, of course, I start to get upset. Frustration and nerves take away my confidence and strength and I falter. Fintan cuts in and says gently, 'If you didn't get upset about this, Janette, what could you get upset about?'

I pull myself together and tell him what we need is a dedicated cancer ward, a ward where admissions and discharges are arranged by our consultants; where beds are solely for cancer patients and are not taken by patients in casualty admissions. We need the closed beds to be opened. Simply put, we need our treatment and whatever must be done to make this happen should be done today. I feel anger at us Irish for being so accepting, for being afraid to rock the boat, to speak out against a government that has the power and the control to make things right for all of us.

I feel pity for those who are without the support of family and friends and have no one to help fight their corner, those who are maybe too weak to stand up for themselves. I try to pack as much as possible into the few minutes but I am weak today. Fintan must sense I am drained and he kindly thanks me and says he doesn't want to add to what must already be a very stressful situation. Next on the line is Dr Carney, an oncologist and, I am happy to say, the consultant who looks after me. He is a person who cares, a genuine, compassionate heart and a man who I feel sees us all as individuals and who treats me and my family with the utmost respect and care. He talks of his battle of eleven years for beds, his agitation that there is an internal struggle between consultants for these hospital beds and how the closure of beds by government some years back is the main reason patients like me are suffering in this way. He tells honestly that my intensive chemotherapy must be given urgently and on time. Even though I know this to be the case his words frighten me and I worry for my life.

The programme goes to an ad break. I am still listening by phone and a researcher asks if I would still like to stay holding. I ask about Michael Martin and if he is still coming on air. She tells me he has been delayed but that they still hope to have him on the show. I hang on – I am afraid I will miss something. Fintan comes back on and introduces our Minister for Health, Michael Martin. The minister admits there is a bed shortage problem but claims that €x billion has been invested and more is to come. Fintan ignores his political response and puts it to him that Foot and Mouth was an animals' disease and yet urgent and immediate action was imposed to handle the situation. He asks why humans must suffer at the hands of the government and says that I am only one in thousands who are suffering because of this bed shortage. The minister must feel trapped, as he reverts to the usual line: 'There are also lots of patients who are cared for and treated very well in the system, Fintan.' I want to scream, 'That's brilliant and that's the way it should be, but we are talking about us, about our life or death, about this nightmare situation we are trapped in.' I hear the minister's exasperation as Fintan continues to grill him about the failing health service, about plans, strategies, committees etc. which seem to delay something that should be sorted now to end the torture for patients. The minister says adding to the problem is an increasing population and an ageing population. These issues are putting extra pressure on the system. My mind is conjuring up sarcastic responses: 'Well wasn't it bright then to go and close beds? Was there no foresight?' 'Oh and sorry, Minister, for getting sick.' 'Tomorrow I will have my granny send a written apology to you for growing old.' I boil with irritation. I just can't understand why everything takes so long, why Dr Carney has battled on for eleven years about this problem and why no urgency seems to surround this issue.

Why will they not listen to us, the patients, to the doctors, to the nurses when we tell how we are all suffering? Why all these years wasted? I just cannot make sense of it.

I finish the interview and try to relax, breathing deep. My face and neck burn red. A rash of nerves covers my chest. I try to calm my body from its fear. I delay, stalling, taking my time shuffling to the ward. I feel my bed is hundreds of miles away. I am greeted on the corridor by a torrent of words – words of support and 'well dones'. We all wander back to the ward together. I crawl to my bed. The weakness consumes every bone and stress eventually has its way. I am wrecked. I can't help wondering if the Minister is also getting slaps on the back and accepting 'well dones' and I worry for this country when I realise in truth that, yes, he probably is.

Looking Forward

Today is the day

Every thought, every breath I have taken for the last six months has all been with this day in mind and I feel so nervous. I want you to understand exactly what I feel: try to think of every exam, every interview, the car crash you had, the day you told your love the spark had gone, the day you broke your parents' hearts. Now think of your gut nerves, think how your head and body felt, think of every time your tummy churned with nerves, think of when your loves have ended and the loss you felt, think of the dark alley and the fear of being alone – now multiply that by a million and you still have no idea of how I feel about today. Today my final scan results are ready and my family and I are meeting with my doctor. The truth is to be revealed; the conclusion one way or another. I struggle to keep my mind focused on now, on this moment, not four hours' time. I try not to conjure up different scenarios in my mind. I refuse to play games in my head. A battle of sense goes on in my brain.

***

What will I take from this whole experience? What feelings will stay with me forever? Will I get to pick and choose? Or will this choice be taken from me and be decided in some nerve cell deep in my brain that, once activated, can never switch off? I want to keep the memories but I want to lose the sadness. I want to remember the illness but I want to lose the fear. I want things to return to normal. I want to have a pain without worrying myself to death and I want to move on, as far away as possible, so far that I can never return to this place. I want to obliterate the feelings that hang like a gloom in the pit of my stomach and soul, and fill me to the brim with worry. I want to be me as I was before. But I am not a fool. I know that will never happen. I have changed and, for better or worse, there is no going back. I know I will be strong and move on. I know I will need my friends and family now more than ever. Because if I am well, I can be weak. Now I can let my guard down. Now I can cry. Now I can have negative thoughts. And they will flow and I will let it all go and I will live again.

***

A family united
We are told to meet at my doctor's office at three and my family are welcome. My family had their own meetings along the way and then the information would be brought to my bed. Talk of trips to America if I need treatment or a hospital bed not available here, talk of trips to anywhere in the universe if it would help. A family in panic trying desperately to leave no stone unturned, internet searches for insight and understanding. I knew I only had to say the word and I would be taken wherever my heart desired, Lourdes, Medjugorje, wherever I felt there might be hope.

***

I am terrified to near numbness and the words of one doctor ring in my ears: 'Your consultant will meet with you when you have your final scan and then he will decide what further treatment might be necessary, i.e. bone marrow transplant, more chemo, radiotherapy, who knows? You will just have to wait.' And so I wait, week in, week out. We all wait, filled with fear, stress and confusion, and all to get here to this time, here to this day and here it is: the outcome.

We meet at my brother's home on North Circular Road and we try to form a list of questions. We are lost; there is no list for the unknown. We sit chatting, trying to pass the time, wishing we could manually change the clocks and the world's time would change with us. We drive the journey, a convoy of anxiety.

I feel my stomach turn. I feel tired, weak and drained with worry. I think of those who have taken this journey alone without the support of a family and I feel blessed to be this lucky. At stages in the car I feel I will definitely pass out. What if the news is bad? My world of positivity, my world of belief could slowly crumble. All my trust in St Anthony and my true faith in myself and God that I would be well could vanish in one negative sentence. Now I would know if it were all a load of rubbish.

The end is nigh

The time comes and we enter the doctor's room. He stands to greet us, all eleven of us, and is genuinely shocked as the mass of bodies squash together in his tiny office. He is a friendly, no-nonsense man and cuts to the chase. He seems to stall and shake his head. My heart pounds – she is running scared again and I pity her. I am staring so hard my eyes feel the strain. I hang on every word, every gesture he makes.

The room is silent as though God speaks. It is as though we are afraid to breathe in case we might miss something. He speaks the words too slowly for our waiting hearts and, it seems, with an edge of disbelief: 'Well everyone, the scans are clear.' We exhale in unison, a breath of relief. It releases the stress of months of waiting, the torture, the hell. And now I am free, I am healed, I am whole again.

Everyone cries and smiles. The biggest smiles, real smiles, the ones I have missed for months and I smile from inside out. No more plastic smiles. No words have been invented to describe how I feel. Joy, happiness, ecstasy, over the moon, elated – words devoid of the real emotion I feel today. It is so much more. I sit rigid, as though glued in position. I watch my family take turns at shaking the doctor's hand and worry he may find himself in A&E with a dislocated shoulder.

Things calm a bit and I try to soak in the news:

'Well, have you any questions, Janette?'

'Yes, I have.' I hear my voice say, 'Why did I get it in the first place?'

The room goes silent as he replies, 'We don't really know. It is not hereditary that we know of. Some studies claim it is environmental; some people who work with chemicals or fertilisers have been known to get it.'

I speak again, 'Will it come back?' And I wonder in silence how many times he has had to answer these questions.

He replies with honesty and, I feel, a little regret, 'I can't say.'

Well, what more do I want? After all, he is not God; he is just a man.

***

Finding my way back

I am consumed by weakness, drained of all my strength, as though I have used every reserve and have nothing left. The war is over; now I must make peace. I have little will but as I continue in my counselling I am learning how to move on, how to take control of my life again. Deep down I know I'll find the will, I have to believe things will be okay. But it's hard to rebuild your life and watch as the circle of support slowly ebbs away, the big fear for everyone around me who cared has been lifted and now I am in remission. I feel lost, dishevelled. Where do I begin? How can I rebuild, fit in? I know it must be this way; life must go on. I must learn how to live again. I must learn to be strong again and I must learn to forgive God, whoever, for the loss of lives, loss of time and the pain, hurt and fear endured by us all. I must try to leave my worries behind and start afresh. And I must learn to stop the anger.

***

A strange gratitude

The sun rays from a cloudless blue sky. I sit enjoying a picnic by Blessington Lake with my parents, sisters, brothers, nieces, nephews, my son Graham, his girlfriend Alison and, of course, my partner Declan. All the gang are here. We are a scatter of bodies spread along the lakeshore, the younger ones supervised as they search the lakeshore with nets for a tiny catch. Some of the girls huddle together on blankets while further along some of the teenagers fish contentedly, their roguish laughter carrying along the shore to our ears. As I observe all this I feel overcome, overcome with gratitude to my cancer. I know that sounds mad but I am grateful for the lessons it has taught me, for the way I now relish every day, especially days like today when I feel a peace and calm in my heart. Cancer changes everything, like these lazy summer days with sunshine beaming on my face, days filled with fun and joy of family and friends. This sad joy grips me. It catches me and drives through me an overwhelming, indescribable feeling of utter gratitude for life. It makes me turn from those I love as tears well in my eyes with the knowledge of the loss that was so close, the escape I have made and the memory of the desire that burned in my being to be here. I thank God I had the strength to keep sight of my goal to be doing what I am doing today and every day, living.

This all-consuming recognition of intense gratitude that I assume will stay forever presents itself when I am at my most content and enjoying life to the full but likewise it grips me when I complain, when I moan, when I forget how wonderful this life is and how unbelievably lucky I am. Just the other day I sat sweltering in the car, stuck in Dublin city traffic. A moment of aggravation gripped me and I became irritated at the city heat and I forgot. How could I forget how I had fought, how I had sweltered on a hospital ward for months wishing every minute the nightmare would end? I scold my mind for its ungrateful, selfish mood. But I am human and I will slip. I have my bad days when I want to be cranky, when I want to have a whinge, but I do it with such guilt and I berate myself afterwards.

Fear of a nine-letter word

Something I find ironic: I am still avoiding saying the word 'remission'. For some reason this nine-letter word frightens me. I decide to dispense with my ignorance and consult the English dictionary. Here we go, a definition of 'remission': 'Reduction in the length of prison term.' How apt! It's amazing – I did get parole after all. Is that not strange? So all this time when I have been asked, 'So how are you? Have you finished all your treatment? Are you clear?' I have been afraid to use that stupid little word. Why? I should be grateful that my sentence has been reduced, but in terms of illness, is that what remission means? Of course not, it means 'easing of intensity'. So this clarity has made me even madder. Here I am telling everyone I am clear – obvious denial on my behalf, or is it?

Maybe not: I believe I am clear, clear from pain, treatment and the hospital; clear from any sign of cancer and the way it showed itself in my body. So, yes, I am free and clear and in remission. REMISSION. It has haunted me for months now and I have been refusing to acknowledge it, even when it shoved itself constantly in my face, laughing from the pages of a doctor's letter produced when I wanted to travel abroad and needed to prove the status of my health. A letter required to reassure some stranger in an insurance company that I would be around for a little longer, that I would not cost them a fortune. God forbid I might take a sudden attack of cancer and die on the plane or by the pool. For whatever reason I fear the word. I am reminded now of the early days when cancer was the word I feared to speak; now I battle with 'remission', a word I feel resembles limbo.

***

Trying to fit in

I have not been out with friends in months. It is as though my social life has been on hold. I like a few glasses of wine or an Indian beer, whatever my fancy on the night. But through fear now I abstain. I am afraid to drink with all the medication and the weakness. I suppose I also worry that if I found some form of repose in it or some comfort in every swallow I might not escape its clutches. On this occasion I decide to go to a friend's house, against my better judgement. It is a big decision, not taken lightly. I know I am weak and my mind is fragile but I want normal, I want to have a bit of craic and be among friends. However, I could kick myself for not heeding my own warnings. My friends sing and party until the early hours, like I used to. I stay up as long as I can but gradually the consuming tiredness has its way and I give in and go to bed around 12.30. Declan lies beside me snoring, content after his

few beers. I lie, weak and ill, staring into the darkness, angry
at myself for putting myself in this situation. I am not able for
this, but sure I knew that before I came. Have I learned
nothing? What about all the new ways of thinking, listening
to your body, minding yourself stuff? What a fool I am. As the
torturous hours pass in agitation I hate myself, lying useless
with no energy, afraid to even drive the journey of darkness
that will take me home, home to peace and sleep. The noise
filters through the floorboards, the music, laughter and voices
– all, it seems, amplified to my ears. My friends have no idea
what it feels like for me – the fear, the draining feeling every
second getting worse and worse, needing so much to rest but
the noise depriving me of sleep. I feel I will truly be found in
the light of day in a coma or dead.

I shake Declan, 'Declan, wake up, I feel awful and I am
scared I might faint.' He squints at me through tired, irritated
eyes, 'What? What's wrong?' 'Sorry, Declan. It's three o'clock
and I can't sleep and I feel really weak and sick.' He gawks at
me, 'What do you want me to do? Neither of us can drive.
You're too wrecked and I've had a few drinks. Do you want me
to ask them to turn it down a bit?' 'Please Deck, just tell them
I am sorry, I need to sleep.' He leaves the bed with a sleepy,
dopey head on him. I hear muffles as he relays the message. I
hear a door close and I listen as the music is turned down a
notch. He returns. 'Thanks, Declan, any problem?' He yawns
and replies, 'No, now let's get some sleep.' I snuggle against his
back and feel my eyes droop, thank God. I am just in sleepland
when a door bangs and a screech of laughter breaks the quiet.
I hear the music turn as loud as before, the singing begins in
unison and I resign myself to a draining, sleepless night.

The next day I wake torn between just wanting out,
wanting to run to avoid any form of conflict and the burning
desire to scream at them, 'You are supposed to be my friends,
for God's sake. I would never do that to you!' I make the
sensible choice and I leave as soon as good manners allow. I

come home and sleep for most of the day and wake hating the new me who couldn't even enjoy a party. I hate the tiredness. I am not prepared for this. However, I remind myself of the lesson learned, a valuable lesson not to be ignored again. Mind yourself. You must take control of your own life or you will be sick again.

Six months on

I look in the mirror; my hair is now a mass of tiny curls replacing my once poker-straight hair. I remember nights as a teenager longing for curls, trying tongs, curlers – anything to make an impact. All the layers of spray only ever held it in place for an hour, maximum, and then it would return, defiant, to its normal, natural strands. I remember as a child I had sometimes been teased and called Cleopatra. Now I see Ronald McDonald reflecting from the mirror – how I have changed! I will not moan; I am glad to have my crowning glory back, no matter what colour, style or shape. I move to my face, still bloated from the constant daily intake of steroids. It is a distortion of what was me. I stare now at my chest and neck, and I see my scars, three in total, engraved forever, a constant reminder for the rest of my life of this terrifying thing that has happened, a thing that could happen any day. I look at the whole scene; I see my chest rise and fall, and I look at life and I smile. How lucky am I.

Lasting memories

Our senses are one of the greatest gifts to be given in this life. It's as though they control the moments that are there forever in our brains, bringing recollection and a flooding of memories. They can bring such joy but then also they can betray us, draw us in without warning or choice, to a place of worry and fear. They invade our memory, looking for recognition and then transport us on a wave of sadness. There are a few culprits I have learned to recognise, the pleasing intruders I accept gratefully, like the smell of Hawaiian Tropic. I have used it for years as a sun screen. One sniff and I can feel the warmth of the sun, the pleasure of relaxation consumes my body and I go into longing for endless flip-flop days without a care in the world. The smell of butter-coated new potatoes, burnt and crispy, and I am wrapped in the warmth of childhood joy – I could be standing in my grandmother's kitchen, cosy and content. It can be heaven. And then like a lash of a whip my senses can be consumed by the smell of a perfume or the sound of a song and with no option I am there, back in time, in a place I don't want to visit. It is as though a list has been etched secretly in my senses. I am oblivious to these invaders until they pounce on my unsuspecting mind and I feel denied control. I have begun to recognise a few of the culprits: cream crackers and Laughing Cow cheese, our little snack with our hospital evening tea; prunes, a necessity as the chemo jams our bowels, sometimes bringing them to a halt; hygiene wipes, our personal protection from germs as our immune system depletes and we become increasingly susceptible to germs and bugs, their smell and the memory can turn my stomach; warm drinking water, left lying stagnant for hours in a jug by your bedside; U2's song 'Stuck in a Moment' – it can reduce me to tears in a second, if I let it. I could be driving along listening to the radio and end up a sniffling fool. These are silly things that remind me of cancer and forever without choice will probably always be there etched in my memory. And they will always be linked to cancer, to fear and it will stay this way, I assume, until the day I die.

***

A year on and still so ill

I have the blues. They have descended on me like the locust to a crop. They are dragging me down so far I fear I will never get up and yet I try to fool myself – I can do this, I am so strong. I have beaten cancer for God's sake. What could be worse? I am Super Woman. But eventually I must acknowledge the truth. I need help and I must be strong enough to ask for it. I return to visit Arc House. I remember going in with the stomach-churning feeling of impending doom, that empty pit hungry feeling that comes with apprehension even though you have eaten for Ireland in your nervous build up. But I have accepted that I need their support again if I am ever to be well. I find I am impatient with the world. I want so much to keep all the goodness that had filled my heart when I was ill. I want to hold the joy, the gratitude for life, the love for life. I want to change and now here I am, angry, guilty and miserable, when I know how much this life means to me, when I have begged St Anthony to save my life, when so many have prayed for my life and now here I am unable to live, unable to move on, to forgive, to rid my mind of guilt, guilt that I live, when so many died.

***

Getting my act together

I am now two years cancer free and have had months of counselling, something I think I would have gone insane without. There was so much inside me that needed to be voiced: anger, sorrow, guilt – oh, and a truckload of fear. I was trying to get on with my life but all was not well. My cancer may have gone but it had made me ill in another way. My tolerance level had dropped; I was angry and I was very afraid of every little pain. Even a headache if it was bad enough could spark fear. I was so angry that most of my hospital friends were dead. I was to find out later I was also feeling very guilty that I still lived. Something had to be done if I was to live my life with any sort of inner peace.

The first day I went to counselling I think I just cried for the hour. I was so embarrassed by this that I never wanted to go back there again. Somehow over the years I had prided myself on being someone who seldom cried. I held this attribute in the highest esteem, but God I really needed to cry now. My brain was so trained, my mind so controlled, the tears had battled their journey. Pride spoke words of guilt to stall the spills of pain pouring from my eyes: 'What right have you to cry when Karen, Patricia, Lucy, Theresa, Susan, Eithne, Rita, to name but a few, have all passed on? How dare you feel sorry for yourself?' I would actually tell myself to cop on and get my act together. It was all so frustrating. I continued going to relaxation classes but avoided making pals with any more people. The sight of a bandanna or wig meant fear and loss, and I just couldn't handle it any more – I was overflowing with my own. I couldn't see my way out. I was in the deep, dark hole in the ground and I hadn't even died. I needed space. I wanted to move on and hated the sad stories. I was consumed by guilt as my hair began to grow. With my treatment ended and no more hospital stays, I saw the envy in the eyes of others who still had a battle ahead. I remember when I felt this jealousy, the wanting burning a hole in my soul and time the enemy. I knew how they were suffering and I felt for them. I had lost so much dignity and confidence with hair loss and cancer.

But counselling made me confront the ache that was burning inside me, to face the anger and frustration that was steaming in my brain. It took me a long time to cry again but eventually my counsellor helped me. As I voiced my fears I felt confident I could learn to live again. I still often remember all the wonderful people I met. I think of their families and know how they suffered, but I just know their spirit lives on and they are at peace. I remember them as brave, strong women and men, facing the end of their lives with dignity and pride and I will hold this memory forever.

Most of the women I knew had no fear of death. They feared for the family and friends they were leaving behind and how they would cope and, yes, they were very sad for what they would never get to experience, the things that seem our right in life but can be taken from us in one missed breath. For some it was the chance of meeting someone, falling in love, maybe getting married, becoming a mother; for others it was missing out on their children's lives, missing all the special times, the ones we take for granted, never for one moment doubting our absence in these precious milestones of life.

I was terrified for my son, as he never had his father in his life and my parents are getting older. Although my family is large and he has lots of cousins, he would have no one to call his own, to understand his humours and his ways like I do; no one to be his Mam, to love him as only a mother can love her child. I write these words always worrying I will offend someone, but they are my thoughts. My partner Declan loves my son very much and I know he would never want for a friend, but it is not the same. These thoughts for me are the most unbearable.

Some women knew they would never have the chance to hold a grandchild, see a child marry. These were the things that mattered. Just wanting to be back on the path life seemed to have chosen for you, never having expected to travel this new one of torment and loneliness. But they knew they would accept their lot and, if nothing else could be done for them, hoped that the end would be fast and painless. The fear is not of death, but of leaving, just not wanting to go. When the ultimate fear stares you in the face what else can frighten you? It has happened, the worst-case scenario, and there is not one thing anyone can do.

***

Days of joy three years later

There are memories in my life that I keep alert and waiting, stored in the forefront of my brain to be churned out at a moment's notice; the feel-good memories that bring peace and quiet to your heart. One of them was made last week. It is three years since I was diagnosed. I was due in the hospital for my usual tri-monthly check-up and I forgot to go. How could I forget? Simple, I put a wrong date in my head. The fact that I actually did this was exciting for me. No, I haven't lost the plot. They say time 'stands still for no man' and yet I felt I had been stuck in Groundhog Day for years. Memories of my illness were always just a touch away; like a person with a compulsive disorder, I had to check my appointment card on a regular basis, just in case. To be honest, by the time my appointment would come I usually had some little worry, so I would be counting the days. There were two reasons I was happy about this lapse of memory: firstly, it meant that I had been very well for the three months and, secondly, that I had relaxed and forgotten about my illness.

And then today the icing on the cake. I attend the hospital this morning, just the regular mundane stomach-wrenching visit, and life changes again. My path is altered by a few simple words. They are totally unexpected and send my head in a spin. It is decided that because I am over three years in remission and because I have been doing so well I will only be having one more scan. I greet this with mixed emotion. Declan's response is instant and one of relief, as happiness beams from his face. My emotions are in a knot.

I breathe, pause and then decide to speak the words I have never dared utter before: 'So am I in the clear?' And his reserved response, 'Well let's say you're more in the clear than in remission.' A very clever man, my doctor, giving nothing away. He leaves the room saying, 'See you in four months!' I look to Declan, his eyes filled ready to spill and I speak quickly, 'Stop, stop, you will start me off.'

You see, I am already thinking ahead to our exit from this room, where at any time at least thirty faces look up to view your expressions as you leave, looking as I have often done, trying to read from the face the news it bears. I remember Trisha, another friend, her eyes burning, red face contorting in pain, I couldn't bear to look. I had spoken to her before she went for her results, nervous, stupid words, 'Please God you will be fine, there is still hope', and I uttered a quick prayer to God that my words would be true. And then I saw her leave. I ignored her, unable to witness her pain, her face distorted, a blur, as my eyes filled. She left supported by her Mam. Her pain real and true.

No, I cannot leave with tears to see the waiting heads bow, misreading the signs and in their misunderstanding feeling my pain, feeling my sorrow and all the while pleading to God it will not be them. No, I could never do that. I will save my tears of joy until I am away from this place. What right do I have to stir thoughts of worry and fear when all the while I am bursting with delight? And while I dress I spare a thought for the next patient, waiting nervously for their life-altering news.

The idea of no scans is a double-sided sword: it is great that it is another step forward but I am also afraid. How will I know if the intruder returns when even the experts failed me in a diagnosis and, unfortunately, as much as I would love to, I can't see through my body? However, it is time to remember what I have learned. My body will tell me if I listen. If I heed its warning I should have some hint if anything ever goes wrong again.

These hospital visits have always brought me a comfort. It's my back-up. The supervisor of my health, overseeing, guarding, ready at hand should any signs show that I am ill again. The blood test, the physical check and mainly the scans are all proof that I am well, the conviction I needed to eradicate the niggles of worry which laze in the corner of my brain. How will I be without these assurances? One more scan, that's all, for, as the doctor says, it's just unnecessary radiation when things are continuously okay. To hear the desired results once more – this time I will listen more closely, engrave them in my brain, 'Scans are clear, guys'. These words are so precious but they roll from his lips so casually. I wonder has he any idea how we all scan his face the minute we see him, watching for a sign, good or bad, a gesture? Would we even know if it showed? Please God, I never have to find out.

***

A glass of wine too many

Today I live. My eyes water involuntarily. I live, it is all I desire. I walk. I stand. I talk. It is real and it is life. I am! I wake each day. How lucky am I? I cry with pleasure in the rain, as it sprays its life on my body; it is pure, real nature; inconsiderate, but real and true. The sun shines, I cry. It shines on a crazy, violent world. I am alive. I feel the heat. I am here. Lucky me. The snow falls. Nature takes no instruction. It is the one, the beginning and end. No kings, politicians; no master or mistress. Yet it rules and we have no say. And we obey. I live and I feel every moment. I will never just be. I will always be grateful, happy, ecstatic, euphoric that the most special gift in the entire world goes on and I am part of it all … Life!

***

Life goes on

Three years on and I feel more like my old self now. I know I will never fully be the person I was before. I am changed forever – cancer does that. I am, I hope, a stronger, braver person, a better person. Never for one minute do I take my life for granted. I can still see the faces of all my hospital friends who were not as fortunate as me and it still upsets me greatly that they had to die. I am so lucky that, for whatever reason, God decided to give me another chance. I will be forever grateful. I was blessed I had so many people's prayers; neighbours, friends, family, people I had never even met prayed for me and I had so much love and kindness bestowed on me. I will always be grateful to everyone who helped me through this time of my life, for without them I know I would not be here. I feel unbelievable appreciation for the nurses in the hospital, my doctor and all his team, and I wish them many blessings and good health. These words seem so insignificant – how do you thank those who saved your life?

Sometimes I see some of the other women from the hospital who, like me, were lucky to survive. Hair grown back, wigs and bandannas a thing of the past. I see their faces glowing with health and happiness reflecting in their eyes. We look at each other wondering, I know that face, but how? And later I remember it. But in a different way; pale complexion etched with worry, devoid of eyelashes or eyebrows, not a hair in sight, face swollen out of its natural shape from medication and I smile to myself and I thank God for our lives and hope we all stay well.

Today I can say that it was worth baldness, vomiting, diarrhoea and insanity – everything, just to be here with my family and friends and to live. 'Oh yes to you wonderful life.' Of course I wish it never happened, but that is life too, and maybe some day I will know why.

I hope my story enlightens you; I hope it makes you angry; I hope it makes you want to do something positive, something in memory of all our brothers and sisters who have left this world. We can still help those who today are battling cancer and other long-term illnesses; those weak and vulnerable, still suffering the indignities and appalling conditions. We need to speak out, we need to stand up and rock the boat. We need to demand changes that can make us proud of our health service and our government. They are all accountable for the suffering of patients; we are all accountable and unless we do something we are not only failing each other, we are failing ourselves.

Is it happening again?

I remember one night sitting with Graham, Alison and Declan, it was like any other night, chilled out watching telly. I don't even know why, but I found my hand rubbing my neck and there it was, a lump, a simple little cluster beneath my skin. Three years on and the fear was as immense as ever. I panicked and uncontrolled, instant tears went running down my face. My family turned to me in confusion, shocked, kneeling beneath me, a circle of fear, faces masked in concern, as I spluttered and slobbered my discovery, crying over and over. 'I can't go through it, I can't do it all again.' We arranged a visit to the hospital for the earliest appointment, which was three days' time. Each day was like a year. We all carried on with pretence at indifference. At this stage we had become experts. I greeted the day of my hospital visit with a churning stomach. It is a strange feeling, the desire to know and the longing to run as far away as possible. I cursed my discovery and damned the lumps to hell and still they stayed.

As usual my doctor treated my concern with compassion and with a desire to ease my worry. Blood tests were ordered and I was told to come back in two weeks to see if the lumps had changed. It was suggested that it could be just swollen glands and a sign I was coming down with something. The following days I waited in terror – a wait like that of the much-wanted missed period – and I begged God that all would be okay. And eventually I was greeted with a welcome smile, a throat infection and some miserable bug. I was never so happy to be sick. The illness passed but the lump stayed, small, but menacing. I still monitor its existence. I remain well and I thank God every day for this chance to live my life.